THE EXPERT WITNESS

Examinations of crimes, drugs and poisons by a forensic toxicologist

William J. Allender

NEW HOLLAND

Dedication

Dedicated to the victims of the crimes and their families, and the police officers and colleagues I have had the privilege of working with on these, and many other cases.

Contents

Introduction

I'm waiting outside another cold sandstone court, its slate roof tiles encrusted with the accumulation of lichens from many years, to present my scientific evidence in yet another drug- and/or poison-related matter and to face the intense scrutiny of the legal process. The greater part of any forensic science investigation involves waiting ... and waiting, whether it's to gather further evidence to put together a brief (I've often marvelled at this word 'brief', which seems to be an oxymoron for the voluminous quantities of papers needed to present a case to court: statements from witnesses, police and victims, plus laboratory reports etc.) or to present my findings. But hopefully, when all of the evidence has been presented and due justice prevails, it will all have been worthwhile. Sadly, however, this isn't always the case.

Poisons and drugs, gathered from a variety of sources, have been used in an illegal way for centuries, and they command an unfortunate, enduring fascination. People appear to be both attracted by them and, at the same time, repelled by them due to the fact that they are not only deadly, but can also be very discreet. Forensic investigations usually give rise to the following questions: Did the victim overdose? What was the poison/drug used? Was it murder, an accident or suicide? How was it taken and in what quantity? Would that dosage be enough to take their life? But in the end, the difference may come down to how it was administered, the probable dosage, the levels of the poison/drug found in the body, the tolerance of the body – and then, the motive for carrying out the deed. As Forrest Gump said in the 1994 movie of the same name: *'Life is like a box of chocolates, you never know what you're gonna get'*. And so it is with many criminal cases: some are darker than others, but none are ever sweet!

This book contains a selection of case stories (some names have been changed for legal reasons) taken from the many I've been involved in over the years. I hope you, the reader, find them both interesting and informative.

William ('Bill') J Allender

MSc; PhD. FRACI; FACBS

Forensic Medical Scientist/Toxicologist

1

A Cry in the Night

'Nobody ever forgets where he buried a hatchet.'
~ Kin Hubbard

In the quiet rural town of Uralla, the cold bleak evening of Saturday, 10 June 2000 didn't promise anything out of the ordinary. And why would it? The last piece of real excitement seen in the sleepy hilly area in the Northern Tablelands of the New England region of New South Wales had taken place some hundred and thirty years earlier when Frederick Ward – aka Captain Thunderbolt, the notorious bushranger – had been shot by the police on 25 May. Situated halfway between Brisbane and Sydney, the 2300 people who inhabited the town went quietly about their business, totally unconcerned with the world outside.

But that tranquillity was about to be disturbed.

At 8.40 pm, the phone in the local police station rang. The caller said, 'I'm from Queen Street. There's some sort of commotion going on at the flats next door. Could you come and check it out?'

A police unit went to investigate and found Marion Read (often called

Mary) and a young female companion shivering outside a flat. Leo Hunt, part Aboriginal and also known as 'Snow' because of his pure white hair, was standing inside by the sliding glass door. The police ushered Marion back into the flat.

'What's going on?' one of the police officers asked.

'Snow assaulted me', Marion replied.

Further conversation ascertained that both parties had been drinking, something which had made for an uneasy relationship between the two in the past. Then Marion said, 'Snow's accusing me of having an affair with the bloke in flat four, but I don't even know him'.

The police officer looked from Marion to a scowling Snow and back again. 'Jealous, is he?'

Marion nodded. 'And possessive.'

'So what happened tonight?'

Marion fixed Snow with a glare. 'He knocked me glasses off me face and forced me up to that bloke's flat, screaming at me. He kicked me and knocked me glasses off me head. I don't even know the bloke in flat four.'

'If you get another AVO (apprehended violence order),' Snow snarled, 'you're dead. I'll fucking kill you'.

'I didn't get the last AVO,' Marion retorted, 'the police did. And for your information, I didn't call them tonight'.

The police officer had heard enough. 'Get up, Snow, and wait outside', he said. Then he turned to Marion. 'Based on what you've told me, I'm going to charge him with assault. I'll be back in a moment.'

An AVO was applied for and subsequently issued by an after-hours magistrate in Parramatta. Its terms were read to Hunt.

'Do you understand all the conditions about not going near Mary?' the police officer asked.

'Yeah, I understand', Hunt replied. 'All this for a fucking 'gin!'

At five minutes to midnight, Snow was conditionally bailed not to approach Marion, who had been strongly warned by the police that she should lock herself in after they left. Unfortunately, she failed to take their advice and, shortly after midnight, there came a knock at her door. Foolishly, Marion opened it. It was Hunt. He forced her back into the flat, but she managed to evade him, turn and run out outside. Hunt picked up a carving knife from the kitchen and gave chase. He was intent on carrying out his earlier threat. Marion ran towards the caravan park, but Hunt was faster and stronger, and he soon caught up with her.

Just forty minutes after he'd been issued with the AVO, witnesses from the nearby caravan park heard a couple of short bloodcurdling screams as Hunt stabbed Marion repeatedly in the back before running off, leaving the carving knife embedded where he'd made his last frenzied thrust.

A few minutes later, the police emergency line received a triple zero (000) call. The caller asked to speak to the Uralla police.

'I can't put you through sir', the operator replied, 'but I can get them to come and see you'.

A short silence followed.

'Hello', the operator said, checking to see if the caller was still on the line.

The caller repeated his request, whereupon the operator repeated what she'd said, adding, 'Or I can get them to contact you by phone'.

The caller then asked the operator to contact the police for him.

'OK', she replied. 'What's your name?'

'Snow Hunt.'

'I'm sorry', the operator said, 'what's your name?'

'Hunt.' Snow also gave his telephone number.

'Can I say what this is regarding, Mr Hunt?' the operator asked.

'What's that?'_

'What is it regarding?'

'I'll talk to the police.'

'OK', the operator replied. 'You don't have an emergency that you need the police to attend to straight away?'

'I think so, yes,' Hunt said.

'You do need the police there straight away?' the operator queried, in an effort to confirm what help was being sought.

'Yes, yes please', Hunt replied

'Well, it's quicker if you give me the details …'

At that point, Hunt terminated the call.

About fifteen minutes later, the Uralla police were contacted. They arrived at Hunt's residence at just gone one o'clock in the morning. The house was in darkness and the front door was closed. A police officer rapped on it sharply, calling out, 'Snow are you in there? What's going on?'

The door opened and Hunt slowly emerged from the darkness. 'What the…?'

'What's going on? Why did you call the cops, talking about Marion?' the police officer asked.

'You obviously don't know what's happened', Hunt replied.

'Where's Mary?'

There was no answer forthcoming, so the police officer repeated his question in a slightly more assertive manner. Hunt stood there for a few moments, but eventually answered, 'In the park'.

'Where in the park?'

'In the caravan park.'

'What have you done to her?'

Hunt stood motionless, saying nothing, but after a few minutes and some further discussion, he led the police to the scene of the crime, where he pointed towards a prone body. 'There she is', he said.

Marion was lying face down in the grass, a large amount of blood around her nose and mouth area, and a large-handled kitchen knife protruding from her back, just as Hunt had left her. A police officer turned to him in despair and anger. 'What have you done?'

'I've had two packets of Serepax [a brand of oxazepam, a benzodiazepine used to treat anxiety and insomnia] and I don't know what I've done', came the reply

'Where did you get the knife?' the police officer asked.

Hunt shrugged. 'What knife? I don't know.'

The police officer then placed Hunt under arrest before cautioning him and putting him in the police car. Then he radioed for back-up. Shortly after, more police and an ambulance arrived at what had been declared a crime scene. The ambulance officer who checked the deceased for any signs of life was also asked to check Hunt because he'd said that he'd taken two packets of Serepax, but the police that had come with the ambulance said that Hunt should go to the hospital. He was taken out of the police car and handcuffed before being escorted to the ambulance, which took him to Armidale Hospital, some twenty-three kilometres away.

In the meantime, the area around the corpse was preserved until crime scene and police detectives arrived, and a search was made of Hunt's premises. Two empty blister packs of Serepax were found. A government contractor showed up after Hunt was taken from the scene and transported Marion's body to Armidale Hospital, where she was formally pronounced dead.

The ambulance transporting Hunt to the accident and emergency section of the hospital arrived at a couple of minutes before two o'clock. The police officers accompanying him reported that he appeared to be alert and orientated, and that there were no other evident problems.

The doctor on duty was briefed on what had happened and, when asked for his version of events, Hunt just said, 'I warned her'.

While hooking Hunt up to a monitor to check his cardiac and respiratory systems, the nursing staff asked the police officer if the handcuffs were really necessary because they were making the task more difficult. By way of an answer, the officer told them that Hunt was alleged to have murdered someone earlier in the evening and that he had taken two foil packs of Serepax.

It was decided to treat him for a drug overdose. Part of the treatment involved the administration of charcoal to absorb the poisons, but Hunt was unhappy with that and objected, saying, 'Do I have to have this shit?'

'Sorry, you have to have it', the nurse replied, matter-of-factly.

Further assessments were also carried out, including the Glasgow Coma Scale (GCS), a test to determine how alert a person is, with a score of fifteen being totally normal. Hunt was assessed as fourteen, and the testing nurse reported that the only area that Hunt seemed confused about was where he was. As far as the nursing staff was concerned, the result of the test showed the oxazepam he had apparently ingested was having a minimal effect at that time, so they asked him what he had taken.

'Two packets of Serepax', Hunt replied.

It was clear from his breath that he'd been drinking, so after a few hours another GCS was performed but, on the second occasion, there was no response to speech or spontaneous action. Judging him to no longer be a threat, Hunt's handcuffs were removed. However, after a final test involving a sternal rub, he awoke and started to throw his arms around, swinging punches at nursing staff, so he had to be re-handcuffed. At the same time he stated to verbally abuse the nurses, saying things such as, 'What the fuck are you doing?'

A further GCS carried out an hour and a half later, at 6 am, rated him as a ten, and he only responded to the sternal rub. Once again, he was released from his handcuffs, but when a nurse attempted to aid his respiration, he suddenly propped himself up on his elbow and said, 'I'm going to kill you', at the same time taking a swing at her. She screamed and colleagues came rushing to her aid, re-handcuffing Hunt once more. It took him an hour to settle down. It was discovered later that he'd developed a tolerance to the oxazepam and had apparently been taking it for many years in an attempt to keep himself calm. Of course, any alcohol in his system would have exacerbated the effects.

Five hours later, at midday, a blood sample was taken. It was found to contain oxazepam 2.2 milligrams per litre (mg/L), which is more than eight times higher than the therapeutic range (0.09 to 0.44 mg/L, average 0.265 mg/L). However, there was no trace of alcohol, even though a witness had said Hunt had smelt strongly of alcohol and had been half drunk. But on the other hand, the witness had also said that Hunt had been talking normally and had had no problems standing up or walking.

Such apparent contradictions can be explained by the time interval between Hunt drinking and having his blood tested - it's probable that any alcohol would have been metabolised to undetectable levels – as Hunt was a regular drinker – and he would have been more tolerant of alcohol and able to metabolise it faster than someone who drank infrequently or just on social occasions.

Marion Reid's post-mortem indicated that she'd had a rough life, with several health problems and a number of bruises of varying ages being revealed. The wounds that most likely took her life were apparent in her chest, and defensive injuries to her hands showed she'd desperately tried to prevent her untimely demise.

Leo 'Snow' Hunt stood for trial on 12 November, 2001, some seventeen months after Marion Reid had been killed. The trial took place in the NSW Supreme Court in Tamworth, where Hunt was charged with his de facto's murder.

I attended Tamworth Court for the committal hearing and gave evidence relating to the level of oxazepam found in Hunt's blood. I was cross examined on a number of issues relating to the drug, including tolerance, absorption time and how long it takes for its effects to become apparent with regard to the quantity taken. For example, if fifty Serepax tablets were taken in one sitting, how would that manifest itself in the stomach?

My answer was that such a large number of tablets would clump together and form a bolus in the stomach and be absorbed over time, the exact length of which would depend on whether food was present. Further questions addressed the possibility that oxazepam ingestion can produce a paradoxical reaction of acute rage rather than sedation. For example, I was asked, from what I knew of the case and based on my knowledge generally, that if one of the paradoxical reactions such as acute rage, stimulation or excitement were to occur, would anything make it possible for that reaction to occur within, say, fifteen minutes of a large overdose of tablets having been taken.

I replied, 'Fifteen minutes seems a bit too fast for me. It would have to be at least a minimum of half an hour. You have to allow time for the stomach to actually absorb the drug into the bloodstream, and you would be still looking at half an hour to an hour for the effects to actually to come into play'.

Both prosecution and defence counsels were basically trying to establish when Hunt took the drug overdose. Was it before or after the murder?

It seemed to me that it was more likely Hunt had taken the drug overdose *after* the murder, possibly in an attempt to take his own life as well. However, even if the drug overdose had been taken just *before* the murder (and there seemed to be no motivation for that), there had been insufficient time for the drug to manifest the various effects put to me, paradoxical or otherwise. That conclusion was borne out by other witness evidence that followed my toxicological evidence.

Hunt was found guilty as charged and sentenced to a minimum of twenty years imprisonment. Given that he was sixty-eight years old at the time of sentencing, it seems likely he'll spend the rest of his life in gaol, while some folk in Uralla will forever be haunted by Marion's agonising cries in the night for as long as they live.

2

A Case of MDMA Madness

'No one other than you yourself is the cause of your ecstasy or agony.'

~ ***Sumit***

MDMA (or 3, 4 - methylenedioxymethylamphetamine) is a popular drug of abuse. Its subjective effects have contributed to its popularity as a party drug among adolescents and young adults who attend rave or rock parties. The drug is mostly smuggled into Australia, although there have been some local attempts to synthesise it. Unfortunately, the local product is gaining popularity due to the perceived notion that the drug is safer than alcohol, but nothing could be further from the truth.

MDMA is a ring-substituted derivative of phenethylamine, which has close structural features related to both amphetamines and hallucinogens, such as mescaline. MDMA is used recreationally for its combination of stimulant and hallucinogenic effects, which combine the effects of mescaline and amphetamine. The drug has no approved medical use in Australia, but is widely abused. It's better known by any one of a variety of street names, including Ecstasy, XTC, Vitamin E, ADAM and even simply 'pills', and the most common ways of taking it are via the mouth (generally in tablet form), by snorting (absorbed nasally), through intravenous injection and as suppositories.

MDMA is rapidly absorbed when taken orally (the usual method of ingestion), while injecting has been reported as having the quickest onset at the same time as producing a more intense, but shorter lasting experience. The effect of taking larger doses is mainly hallucinatory with undesirable side effects increasing in relation to the amount taken. The onset of action is usually within thirty to forty minutes and a maximal response is achieved in about one to two hours. The duration of action is about four to six hours (average five hours) and the drug and its metabolites are excreted mainly in the urine.

The negative effects of ecstasy are dose-related, in that their severity correlates with both the total number of doses consumed and the frequency of use. Short-term high-dose use of MDMA has produced incidences of an amphetamine-like psychosis and, in some cases, severe hyperthermia that was unresponsive to medical intervention, leading to death. It can also cause a paranoid psychosis or chemically induced madness.

MDMA and its congeners constitute potential health hazards of uncertain proportions for human users. Behavioural manifestations of MDMA use are typical and distinctive. They include rapid and confused speech, dilated pupils, agitation, paranoia and a violent, aggressive demeanour. The degree of the effects present generally increases with the blood-MDMA concentration, with violent, paranoid behaviour being attributed to a very high blood-MDMA concentration.

The Big Day Out (BDO) is a cultural event that has taken place every year since 1992, and it's the longest-running and biggest rock festival in Australia. It's travelling circus of nearly one hundred local and international acts play in five Australian cities and Auckland (New Zealand) before a total audience of about two hundred thousand, making it one of the largest rock events in the world. In Sydney, it draws a crowd of fifty-five thousand, and the BDO on 26 January 2001 was no exception. Amongst the featured artists were

Australia's acclaimed Powderfinger, Germany's fire-breathing Rammstein, and the headline act Limp Bizkit, plus five separate rooms of disc jockeys.

During the Sydney gig, a twenty-three-year-old man purchased a quantity of MDMA from an unknown supplier. When the BDO wound down, he went to a friend's house in Neutral Bay where he texted his girlfriend at just gone half past one in the morning to say where he was, and that he was spending the night there before returning home the following day. However, he left the friend's house an hour later, wandering off into the night. After a while his friend, who'd assumed that he would probably return to his place, became worried and tried to contact him via phone, only to receive a mouthful of abuse before the young man hung up. Thinking that the response was out of character, he tried again several times over the next half hour, always without success. At about 4.30 am the young man picked up and told his friend that he was on Sydney Harbour Bridge. The friend wasn't sure what to make of that, but was concerned because, as he told the police later, the young man 'turned funny all of a sudden'.

Shortly after, the young man, under the influence of the MDMA he'd taken earlier, began to cause chaos on the bridge. He started walking down the middle of the road, even trying to jump in front of oncoming cars. The affected motorists called the police and, on one occasion, the young man leapt on top of a vehicle and started kicking and punching it. The police rushed to the bridge at about half past five and attempted to remove him. They got hold of him and were escorting him back to their truck when he began to struggle and fight, causing all parties to fall into the roadway. The police tried to immobilise him with capsicum spray but it had no effect, and as they were attempting to pull him off the road and away from the traffic the young man was struck by a vehicle in the southbound lane. When the ambulance and paramedics arrived at the scene, they found him lying in a pool of blood and, in spite of trying everything they knew, the injuries he'd sustained were too severe and his life just ebbed away. He was taken to hospital, where he was later officially pronounced dead.

At the autopsy, a blood sample taken from the deceased was found to contain MDMA 2.1 milligrams per litre and methylamphetamine 0.3 milligrams per litre. The level of MDMA was particularly high and well within the lethal range. It indicated a very high dosage (estimated at approximately 1 gram of the pure drug ingested orally), and suggested that the deceased had been a heavy user of MDMA, although that may or may not have been true. I suggested that the presence of the methylamphetamine may have been due to either its direct ingestion or that it may have been present in the original MDMA preparation.

The inquest took place on 21 November, 2001, and it was obvious from the outset that the deceased was a popular and much loved young man as friends and family members wept openly during the proceedings, at one time necessitating a brief adjournment so they could compose themselves.

In the witness box, I reiterated much of what I'd said at the autopsy, which was supported by a brief from Professor Graham Starmer, then with the Department of Pharmacology, Sydney University. It was clear that the bizarre behaviour exhibited by the deceased on Sydney Harbour Bridge was well out of character, and was almost certainly caused by the very large doses of MDMA and methylamphetamine. Whether those drugs were mixed together or one was an impurity was not known.

The post-mortem blood levels obtained for both drugs were potentially lethal, more so the MDMA level and, therefore, the collision may simply have hastened the young man's final outcome. However, given the level of the drugs detected, it's possible that if he'd been given rapid medical intervention, he may have survived. Unfortunately, we will never know.

3

The Corpse in the Culvert

'Death is the solution to all problems.
No man – no problem'
~ ***Joseph Stalin***

LSD (lysergic acid diethylamide) gained its notoriety in the late 1960s and early 1970s when it became the drug of choice for the hippie generation. Dr Timothy Leary promoted its allegedly carefree properties in the late sixties with the mantra 'turn on, tune in, and drop out' (of society). Unfortunately the reverse is true, as the drug upsets the brain chemistry of the user resulting in hallucinations and various other behavioural problems, with dreaded flashbacks occurring without the drug even being detected in the bloodstream. In fact, the d-isomer of LSD is one of the most potent hallucinogenic drugs known, and yet it has a remarkably low acute toxicity, with a therapeutic index (therapeutic ratio) in the order of 1000. The therapeutic index is a rough indication of how safe a drug is likely to be – the higher the index, the better - although it isn't the be-all and end-all measure when it comes to safety, and caution must be used when quoting a drug's therapeutic index, as some of our most valuable drugs have low ones. For example, opiates such as morphine and codeine.

LSD is usually taken by drug abusers as a tartrate salt in oral doses of twenty-five to two hundred and fifty micrograms via tickets (absorbent paper containing the drug and also known as trips or tabs), which are often decorated in heart- or geometrical-shaped logos. LSD was originally developed as a clinical drug, but its use was abandoned because of its unpredictable flashback side effects. However, despite its erratic nature, it has maintained as a popular recreational drug.

This story takes place in Wollongong, an industrial town of over two hundred and fifty thousand people on the picturesque south coast of New South Wales. Best known for its iron and steel production at Port Kembla, it also has some beautiful beaches and the escarpment semi-rainforest.

William 'Liam' Tully-Slater was an easy-going, friendly type. Part aboriginal, he believed that friends should share everything - a quality that is nurtured in the aboriginal community, as it can make all the difference between survival and extinction of said community. However, his white-skinned friends took a different view. They considered his taking of food and various other items to be no less than stealing and they were getting fed up with his behaviour, regarding him as a bit of a nuisance. Unfortunately for Liam, he didn't get the message.

On the evening of 15 November, 2000, Liam's friends Jason Farrell, Daniel Ezold, Kai Purhonen and Holly Turner were in a pub, drinking, after consuming a couple of LSD tickets. The conversation turned to Liam and the fact that he was a problem that needed sorting out and, as they talked, a plan to deal with him emerged.

When they left the pub later that evening, they were all intoxicated. Liam, who hadn't been in the pub but had been drinking elsewhere, joined them as they went for a walk to the nearby Tom Thumb Lagoon, a place that Ezold knew well from the time he'd worked in the area as bush regenerator. He'd also once said it would be a good place to get rid of someone. As they strolled, out of the blue, Ezold struck Liam over the head with a Passion Pop bottle, catching him totally unawares. Farrell then grabbed the bottle and continued beating Liam with it, forcing him to the ground, whereupon he kicked him down the embankment and into a stormwater drain near the grain terminal.

Farrell then held Liam's head under the water, saying 'This is how Melbourne boys do it. What's your mother's maiden name?'

Liam wasn't able to respond, only gurgle as he fought for his life. Farrell called to Ezold and Purhonen to help him, which they did, kicking Liam before Farrell pushed his face under the muddy water for the final time, holding him there until he'd ceased struggling and his body had gone limp.

The friends left Liam's body in the culvert and walked to Wollongong beach where Farrell said they should clean their clothing and footwear in the sea to wash away any evidence of the crime. While they were doing that, he said, 'I'm gonna celebrate with some Scotch and a White Owl cigar tomorrow, and I'll top off anyone who talks. I've done a few drownings'.

His meaning and intention were quite clear.

A couple of days passed and Holly felt very uncomfortable with what the group had done. Besides the nagging guilt, she also felt fear lest they should be found out. After two sleepless nights and much internal wrangling, she could stand the torment no longer and contacted the police, telling them, 'There's a young man's body lying in a sewerage drain. Please check it out'.

With the aid of the police rescue squad, Liam's body was promptly found lying face up and partly submerged in the dirty water. A crime scene was established and detectives, including various specialists, were called in to investigate.

Detective Greg Moon from the Wollongong Crime Scene Unit arrived at 7.30 pm on Saturday 18 November. He spoke to Senior Constable MacIver from the police rescue squad and was shown the body, noting that it was dressed in blue, work-type trousers, maroon underpants, brown work boots and brown socks. There was also a t-shirt partially wrapped around the left arm. As for external physical injuries, there were abrasions to the left hand and a small abrasion on the right side of the stomach. Partial rigor mortis was still present in the body, which was covered with dirt and silt, while there was mould around the head and on both sides of the stomach. The dirt and silt on top of the chest had dried.

The police located a number of shoe prints in the nearby sand and mud, including one full set which led right up to the deceased and back again. The shoe prints closest to the body were only just still visible as they had been nearly washed away by tidal waters, eliminating the finer details of the tread pattern, although the remaining shoe prints were clearer, with their tread patterns being distinguishable. There were two further partial marks which appeared to be a different shoe print, one of them being located underneath the other shoe prints, indicating that it had been left prior to the others. Detective Moon later made three plaster cast moulds of the prints.

Having examined the shoe prints, Detective Moon then conducted a presumptive test for blood where the body had been located, using the chemical luminol. Luminol is a chemical used to locate bloodstains that are difficult to see or invisible to the naked eye. When luminol and blood react together, a chemical reaction takes place and blue light is produced. The tested area luminesced.

A green bottle was also seen in the water, but not retrieved until the following Monday, after further information about the case had been received.

Before Liam's body was conveyed to the Wollongong morgue, photographs were taken from various positions and angles and more shoe prints with distinguishable tread patterns were found near the exit of the culvert.

It wasn't long before Jason Farrell, Daniel James Ezold and Kai Purhonen were arrested and remanded in custody and, at 3.30 on Sunday, 19 November 2000, detectives entered a premises on Seaview Avenue, Coniston, armed with a search warrant. The place was very untidy, with clothing and possessions spread all over – a scene of utter squalor. The detectives removed many items of clothing and footwear, all belonging to the three men in custody, and took them to the forensic laboratory.

The following afternoon, tests were carried out on the items, and some dark-red smears were found on the right sleeve of a jacket belonging to Jason Farrell, which tested positive for blood. Shortly afterwards, his boots also gave a positive reaction. The same positive reaction occurred when pants belonging to Daniel Ezold were tested. Evidence was mounting against the pair but, unfortunately, none of the footwear seized by police matched any of the footprints found at the crime scene, although Holly's shoes were later to found to match one of the patterns seen at the scene of the crime, adding some veracity to her 'confession'.

In the meantime, the post-mortem was carried out by Dr Cala and his assistant Dr Sugo at the Institute of Forensic Medicine, Glebe. The report said the cadaver showed evidence of mould on the arms and flanks and moderated decomposition change to the face, neck and upper chest region, although the exact time it was held under the water was unclear. There was, however, a suggestion it may have been as long as five to ten minutes. The lungs were hyper expanded, but there was no obvious fluid in the airways. Such findings were suggestive of, if not diagnostic for, drowning.

After the post-mortem, Detective Moon took possession of the following exhibits and specimens that had been found on the deceased:

- an empty packet of Gitanes cigarettes and a green cigarette lighter collected from the victim's pants,
- a pair of orange secateurs,
- a pair of work boots,
- a pair of socks,
- a pair of blue work trousers,
- a pair of maroon underpants, and
- a 'Quicksilver' t-shirt.
- a sample of blood for grouping,
- an oropharyngeal swab,
- a rectal swab
- his left fingernails,
- his right fingernails,

- some head hair,
- some pubic hair, and
- some sand/grit collected from the deceased's lungs, which indicated the deceased had been alive at the time he'd been pushed into the stormwater drain and that he'd fought for his life in the final minutes before his death and had struggled desperately to breathe minutes before he drowned.

Jason Farrell, Daniel Ezold and Kai Purhonen, all nineteen years old and all of Seaview Road, Coniston, Wollongong, were soon charged with Liam's murder, and the matter subsequently went to court, where the fourth member of the drinking party, Holly Turner, gave vital evidence.

Jason Farrell pleaded not guilty to murder, but guilty to manslaughter on the grounds he was very intoxicated at the time, and the jury subsequently heard that he was 'off his face' on a combination of alcohol and LSD. For the prosecution, evidence was given that Jason Farrell seemed excited over the prospect of having bashed and drowned the deceased, and that shortly after the murder he was high, singing and skipping and making jokes about it. The jury was told how he'd struck Liam on the head with a bottle and then kicked him down the embankment into the stormwater drain before holding him under the water until his face was blue.

When Daniel Ezold entered the courtroom, the jury heard that not only was he a regular drug user, but he also drank daily to excess and was well on his way to becoming an alcoholic. On the night of the murder, Ezold had taken a trip and a half of LSD and had consumed a large quantity of wine. The court was also told that Liam Tully-Salter had been on drugs, too, with LSD being detected in a urine sample taken at the post-mortem and, although he hadn't been with his friends in the pub, he'd also been drinking heavily on the evening he was murdered. As a result, his ability to defend himself would have been compromised. When asked about his actions, Ezold said that he and Tully-Slater had been friends for life and that what happened was just a bit of drunken nonsense.

The defence barrister, Mr Gordon, said the Crown had no reliable evidence that there had been a pact to harm Liam Tully-Salter, even though it had been suggested that one had been formed in the pub on the night the deceased died, with talk of a Musketeer's threesome to carry out the deed. For his part, Ezold told the court that he couldn't recall anything about the death of Liam Tully-Salter and had been shocked when he heard the allegations. 'I'm blown away', he said. 'I don't expect to hear I've been out killing people.'

However, two weeks later, he wrote a letter of remorse and guilt in gaol, detailing his involvement in the murder. In it, he related: *We walked down to Tom Thumb Lagoon because I thought it would be a good place to get rid of someone. I hit Liam over the head with a Passion Pop bottle and kicked him a couple of times.* He also indicated that Farrell, who was apparently the ringleader of the group, grabbed the bottle off him and continued with the bashing until Liam was unconscious. *Don't hate me,* he wrote. *It's not a hard step to kill. I might get off with manslaughter. I didn't actually kill him, just helped with the process.*

Given the amount of alcohol Ezold had already consumed that night, together with the trip and a half of LSD, it was difficult for detectives to discern how he'd been able to help with the process (of murder) unless he'd developed a considerable tolerance to alcohol.

The third co-accused, Kai Purhonen, a Wollongong punk rocker and bass player with the band Blurred Vision, appeared to be in a more complex situation. He was charged with being an accessory to the murder, but was not committed to trial. At the time he wasn't required to enter a plea, as there was doubt about how deeply he'd been involved in the assault which led to Liam's death – he only appeared to have stood by and watched Tully-Salter die. The defence council stated, 'Clearly, he was not at the forefront of this unhappy crime'. Furthermore, he appeared to have been affected by LSD and alcohol at the time of the murder. Nevertheless, Kai Purhonen was kept in custody for nearly eighteen months, waiting to prove his innocence, while Farrell and Ezold were gaoled for eighteen years and sixteen years respectively.

Although the murder had been committed on the evening of 15 November 2000, it wasn't until 3 May 2004 that I, along with Professor Graham Starmer of Sydney University, was subpoenaed to appear in the Supreme Court.

I gave evidence with regard to the effects of LSD on a person's faculties and sensibilities. It wasn't an easy call, as I didn't know whether Purhonen had been a regular user or not. However, some affectation by a drug did seem to be indicated, although he could also have been suffering from other mental problems upon which I was not qualified to comment. After a three-week hearing, the jury took just half an hour to clear Kai Purhonen of murder, rejecting evidence from Holly Turner that he'd been involved in favour of accepting Purhonen's version that he didn't know what was happening until it was too late. Given the quantity of alcohol he had consumed, together with the LSD, I had to agree with them.

That should have been that for Purhonen, as people are usually allowed to go free on the day they're acquitted, but it took another month to secure him Supreme Court bail because of several other outstanding charges, including an incident at the Oxford Tavern where he'd defended himself against taunts and jeers. As a result, he was charged with wounding and his bail was revoked. He then spent the next five months in custody before his murder trial in the NSW Supreme Court. Eventually, the extra charges were finalised in a two-day hearing in Wollongong Court.

Perhaps unsurprisingly, the period of incarceration had a profound effect on his outlook on life. Gaol rendered him withdrawn and depressed. His creativity was sapped by his experiences and he no longer played music. Instead, he fought depression and drank heavily to lessen the pain.

Eventually, the toll of the four years that had passed since the Liam Tully-Salter killing became too much and he committed suicide by hanging. His family was very angry that even his acquittal hadn't ended his ordeal, and they felt he should have been released from prison with some form of support, including counselling and medication. Unfortunately, such a scenario is fairly common for released prisoners, which may account for the re-offenders.

Kai Purhonen went to his grave without any criminal convictions, and funeral attendees were urged to bring a tree to plant in his honour. The whole affair had seen the pointless death of two young people as a result of 'just a bit of drunken nonsense'.

4

No Laughing Matter

'I used to always think that I'd look back
on us crying and laugh,
But, I never thought I'd look back on us
laughing and cry.'
~ Ralph Waldo Emerson

Nitrous oxide has been used in dentistry and medicine for over 150 years. Discovered in 1776 by Joseph Priestly, its potential as an anaesthetic was only recognised twenty-three years later by Humphrey Davy, and it didn't come into general usage until after 1860. Non-flammable and nearly odourless, with a slight sweetish smell, it won't produce complete anaesthesia at safe concentrations (65 per cent oxygen) and so is used mainly as an analgesic (pain relieving) agent in dentistry. It is relatively insoluble in body tissues and fluids and so induction and recovery are generally quite rapid.

It gained its other moniker of 'laughing gas' because of its effects before anaesthesia, when it produces a type of laugh along with a feeling of euphoria.

As a result, it was (and still is) used recreationally at parties in much the same way that ecstasy is used at rave parties today.

It can readily be obtained from medical supplies or whipped cream cans, where it's used as a propellant that mixes in the liquid cream. When the cream escapes from the can, the gas expands and in the process whips the cream into a foam. However, it isn't all fun and games, as the inhalation of 40 per cent nitrous oxide in air causes confusion and sedation, while a level of 80 per cent causes unconsciousness in most people.

In 2000, Dee Why (a coastal suburb of northern Sydney) had, in common with many other towns throughout the country, a church youth group where the young people of the community could socialise in an apparently caring religious setting, watching videos and playing X-box and other games.

One of the youth leaders, a Mr Buggers (not his real name, but one that was deemed to be very apt at the time) took a special interest in the teenage boys in his care, and invited a few of them to his residence on a warm Saturday in August. One of those was fifteen-year-old Scott Evers, who was looking forward to spending some more time with his friends in a relaxed environment. He arrived at midday and knocked on the door. Mr Buggers parted the drawn curtains and peered out. Seeing Scott, he smiled and went to the door, welcoming the boy inside. Two of Scott's friends were already there – but to Scott's horror they were in various states of consciousness and neither was wearing any clothing from the waist down. Scott turned and left, ignoring Mr Bugger's attempts (both verbal and physical) to get him to stay, and reported what he'd seen to his parents, who went to the police.

The police acted swiftly and interviewed Mr Buggers and his victims, in the process uncovering a whole series of sexual abuses and Mr Buggers' *modus operandi*. As a local schoolteacher and church elder, he'd gained a position of trust and authority within the community, which – up until Scott – had deterred his victims from outing him. Being youngsters, they thought that they wouldn't be believed and possibly even be punished for making up stories. Added to that, Mr Buggers also used his position to make credible threats of what might happen to them if they were to tell.

Mr Buggers ran what he called his creaming club, which he set up in order to entice young men ranging from the ages of eleven to twenty-three into being sexual participants. He'd use his many wiles to attract bored or otherwise unemployed males to his home, where he'd administer them doses of nitrous oxide via various whipped cream canisters which had had the cream removed and replaced by nitrous oxide gas bulbs. The young men, promised that it was just a bit of fun, then inhaled the gas. After a brief period of laughter they became semi-conscious, experiencing varying degrees of disinhibition. Unaware of what was going on, or even where they were, they were then sexually abused by Mr Buggers.

Mr Buggers was subsequently charged with a number of offences relating to sexual/indecent assaults upon young male persons under Section 38 of the Crimes Act in that he 'did unlawfully cause to be taken chloroform or stupefying drug or thing to commit an indictable offence'.

One of his victims testified that Buggers done it to a whole range of people and had photos of them on a computer, while another victim said that he'd passed out and when he'd woken up, Buggers had been feeling his private parts. When asked how he felt when he woke up to find Buggers putting his mouth over his penis, he replied, 'I don't know. I felt like I was stoned'. Interviews with other victims were disturbingly similar, with one saying that Buggers had pretty much raped him.

I was asked if I could say, in my expert opinion, that nitrous oxide was a stupefying drug or thing, and was disinhibiting to the user – which I could and did, as did the other experts who were called.

The case may have been about laughing gas, but the judge and jury were anything but amused.

Mr Buggers was sentenced to thirteen years imprisonment, with a non-parole period of nine and a half years, giving him plenty of time to reflect on his former lifestyle and, hopefully, make appropriate amendments. But can a leopard change its spots? Only time will tell.

5

The Westpac Bank Robbery: 'Steroids made me do it!'

'There are some things so serious
you have to laugh at them.'
~ Niels Bohr

On a warm December morning in 2003, five days before Christmas, Susan Aquino – branch manager of the Westpac Bank in Auburn, Sydney – arrived for work as usual just before 8.30 am. Staff rostered to work at the bank that day were already at the front entrance, waiting to be let in. Also present was an electrician to fix an air conditioner. Ms Aquino entered the bank alone and carried out various safety checks on alarms and locks before allowing her co-workers to enter the bank to begin another day's business.

As they filed in, and before she could close the doors again, they were joined by what appeared to be three Telstra workers. At least, that's who they said they were, but the tallest one was wearing an orange safety vest, a straw-style hat, black sunglasses and a white dust mask on his face. His two shorter accomplices also wore orange safety vests, but had white hard hats to accompany their black sunglasses and white dust masks.

Ms Aquino regarded them suspiciously, especially as the tallest of the three showed no personal identification when addressing her. 'We're going to do some work for Telstra and electricity', he said. But whatever suspicions Ms Aquino held, it was too late – the three men had gained entry and they quickly revealed their true motive for being in the bank. The tallest 'worker' told her to close the door, which she did.

'Good. Now all of you come in here', he demanded, talking to the other staff, 'and lie face down on the floor, and stop looking at us. We want the ATM money. Who's in charge here?'

'It's me', Susan Aquino replied in a calm voice.

'Then open the ATM', the tall robber growled.

'I can't, because I don't have the combination', Ms Aquino stated.

'Why's that?' one of the shorter robbers asked, waving a Taser menacingly in his hand.

'The girl who does it isn't here today. We don't open them on the weekend. As she spoke, Ms Aquino surreptitiously reached for the silent alarm button under the desk.

'Alright then, we want the treasury money', the tall robber barked, producing a 9mm Luger pistol from his pants.

Anger, confusion and a sense of humiliation coursed through Susan Aquino's veins as she looked into the face of the brawny young man. His outfit was farcical, but as he was pointing a gun at her, she had no choice but to obey his orders, no matter how much she detested him and them.

'I'll take you to the main bank safe', she said, a note of resignation in her voice.

Two of the robbers accompanied her while the third stayed behind to bind the hands and feet of the other bank staff with cable ties.

It took a little while, but Susan Aquino eventually found the codes for the main safe, which allowed access to the main money supply (the treasury) held by the bank. The main safe had a time delay, which caused one of the robbers to betray his nerves. 'Are you delaying?' he snarled as he and his colleague took the tellers' money from the other safes and stuffed it into their black bag.

'No', Susan Aquino replied. 'The keys wouldn't fit in.'

Meanwhile, the treasury safe unlocked and, as Susan Aquino opened the door, the tall robber reached in and grabbed hold of a container of money, emptying it into the black bag together with a number of foreign currencies.

Just as the tall robber finished, the walkie-talkie crackled into life with the voice of the third accomplice: 'The cops are outside'.

'Hurry up and open the doors', the short robber said.

Susan Aquino walked to the front of the bank, looked out and, seeing no one was there, pressed the button to release the lock. The robbers ran out, straight towards the police, dropping the black bag on the floor of the bank's entrance. Unfortunately for the police, the three robbers each elected for a different means of escape, with the two shorter ones bolting in opposite directions. The tall robber unwisely chose to rely on the firearm in his pocket to extricate him from the situation in which he found himself.

He started to walk towards the ANZ bank, just down the road. He placed his right hand on the handle of his firearm, then withdrew it from his pants and raised it towards the police. Detective Senior Constable Paul Arnold, quickly recognising the danger to both himself and his colleagues, drew his pistol, yelling out to the robber: 'Put the fucking gun down. Put the fucking gun down!'

The robber looked around. He was surrounded by a number of police, all with their firearms drawn and trained on him. Arnold shouted at him again to put the gun down and, realising he was outnumbered, the robber muttered, 'Aw, shit, shit…!' After a few seconds' hesitation, he dropped his weapon into a nearby garbage bin. Unarmed, he was wrestled to the ground by the police, sprayed with oleoresin capsicum and handcuffed.

The police quickly retrieved his gun, a 9 mm Parabellum calibre CZ manufactured self-loading pistol. The serial number had been removed and there were thirteen out of a maximum of fifteen live rounds in the magazine, indicating that he had clearly meant business.

As police were dealing with him, one of his accomplices was seen getting into a blue Subaru WRX motor vehicle and, after accelerating harshly, he drove south along Auburn Road, causing a number of police to jump out of the way to avoid being run down.

Meanwhile, the third robber ran towards the rear of Coles' supermarket but despite searching high and low, police were unable to locate him. They did find, however, that in his haste to get away he'd discarded a number of items, including a Uniden handheld scanner. The tall robber, whose name was found to be Jamil Jaafar, was taken to Auburn police station where he was electronically interviewed and later charged with a number of offences, including robbery while armed with an offensive weapon.

On 21 June 2004, he was committed at Burwood Court House. Bail was refused and the matter was then committed to the district court in Sydney, eleven days later.

Meanwhile, Jaafar and his solicitor came up with a novel defence for his actions, probably hoping to persuade the judge to only impose a reduced sentence. They even obtained the services of a consultant psychologist and criminologist, Mr Peter Clark-Saunders, to make their case.

Their defence rested on the fact that Jaafar had always been keen to improve his body image. He had been extremely overweight as a child, and so had taken to the gym. However, to speed up his physical development, he'd supposedly embarked on a course of steroids between the ages of seventeen and eighteen.

At the time of the attempted robbery he was nineteen, and his body had been subjected to a variety of anabolic and androgenic steroids to bolster his muscle mass, which his defence argued gave him steroid induced rage. In other words, they were saying that his judgement at the time of the offence had been affected by his steroid use or, to put it another way: the steroids made him do it. Jaafar himself weighed in, saying, 'I was high on steroids and I was out of control'.

It was claimed that Jaafar had injected Sustanon (one of several trade names for testosterone), Stanazole (a trade name for stanozol) and Decka 50 or Deca durabolin (a trade name for nandrolone decanoate) at quite extraordinary levels. The dosages he'd initially used were supposedly the following:

- two hundred and fifty milligrams per millilitre, twice a week (five hundred mg) of Sustanon;
- a hundred and sixty milligrams per week of Stanazole; and
- a hundred milligrams per week of Decka 50.

After six weeks, he raised the levels to eight hundred milligrams per week of Sustanon and three hundred and twenty milligrams per week of Stanazole.

Mr Clarke-Saunders observed, quite rightly, that that amount of intravenous anabolic usage was sufficient to introduce a syndrome referred to as steroid rage, as Jaafar's supposed steroid regime of eight hundred milligrams per week of Sustanon was four times more than the recommended top-end dosage, and the three hundred and twenty milligrams per week of Stanazole was just over twice the level used by athletes who self-administer the drugs to improve their sports performance. Even the Decka 50 at a hundred milligrams per week was three to four times higher than the recommended top-end dosage. If Jaafar's claimed dosages were true, he'd certainly been on a hefty regime, which would have led to serious health problems including oedema (fluid retention and bloating), suppression of clotting factors of the blood, elevated cholesterol (cholesterolemia), mood disorders and depression.

Furthermore, it's likely that the steroids would have been obtained illegitimately which cast doubt on their potency, as such street drugs are not subject to any controls – unlike prescription medicine – and so they are subsequently quite often of dubious quality (unless stolen from a pharmacy), and are frequently adulterated and diluted, generally to improve the profit margin of the drug dealer.

Jaafar stood for trial on 22 April 2005, in the NSW District Court, for armed robbery at the Westpac Bank, Auburn on 20 December 2003. Judge Hosking presided while Ms Natalie Olender was the crown prosecutor and Mr Andrew Bellanto QC appeared for the defence.

Mr Clarke-Saunders was examined at length about the amount of intravenous anabolic usage that is sufficient to induce a syndrome referred to as steroid rage. His Honour further questioned Mr Clarke-Saunders about Jaafar's alleged serotonin deficiency: 'Just so that I understand this Mr Clark-Saunders, are you saying that this man had a serotonin deficiency?'

Clark-Sanders replied, 'It's a hypothesis', going on to say that his experience in the area led him to believe that Jaafar did indeed have such a deficiency.

His Honour continued. 'You've said in your report, under the heading impulse control disorder, "his psychological steroid addiction and associated rage is compounded by serotonin deficiency". The reason I asked you that question is that you seem to state that as a fact, whereas you are now telling me that it is really a hypothesis. Is that correct?'

Clark-Sanders stated that it was his professional opinion.

Further questioning by legal counsel and the judge centred on the clinical depression, impulse control disorders and serotonin deficiencies supposedly brought about by Jaafar's steroid usage. One key question was, 'Are you able to say then how you came to the conclusion that a precipitating factor to the offender's offending behaviour is one of steroid rage if in fact you didn't take a history from the offender in relation to that use of anabolic steroids?'

Mr Clark-Saunders replied that he'd incorporated Internet research from NIDA (National Institute on Drug Abuse) together with research into anabolic steroids and the mind, and he'd come to his conclusion because when he'd reviewed the defendant's history, there'd been no evidence of criminality prior to the current offences. Although he'd been suffering from depression, there had been no history of anti-social behaviour.

I was subsequently called and cross-examined by the defence, being asked '…do you agree that steroid use can affect one's belief in oneself, affect one's behaviour, that type of thing, depending upon dosage?' I had to agree, though I qualified my concurrence by saying it also depended on the dosage because at various high levels there's anecdotal evidence that it can cause mood changes in some people.

On being probed further, I explained the problems associated with steroid usage, particularly the lack of purity with those obtained on the black market.

Further questioning sought to establish a link between steroid usage and rage.

I stated that 'Rage by definition, whether steroid induced or otherwise, is violent, uncontrollable anger'.

It was also put to me, 'You've indicated there from the fact sheet that it doesn't appear that the offender's behaviour in relation to his role was that of any aggressive behaviour'.

I had to agree. Furthermore, not only did the amount and type of steroids he had supposedly taken appear to be very unlikely, given the likelihood of black market origins of the steroids, the purity would have been doubtful. There have been various reports and studies that suggest a link between anabolic steroid use and aggressive behaviour, but a causal relationship has not yet been clearly established.

It may be that people who are potentially more aggressive are more likely to use anabolic steroids, but at this moment in time, despite reports of violent behaviour among steroid users, there appears to be little scientific evidence that use of anabolic steroids actually causes aggression.

It was unlikely that Jaafar was in a steroid induced rage compounded by a serotonin deficiency, especially when you consider the facts that the robbery was planned meticulously down to the last detail, the staff were carefully restrained with cable ties, Uniden handheld scanners were used, staff were threatened with Taser stun guns and previous inside knowledge of banking practices was used to the robbers' advantage. Without doubt, it was a well-organised and professional robbery, and but for the swift action of Susan Aquino in pressing the silent alarm button, it's probable that Jaafar and his accomplices would have escaped with a very large amount of stolen money.

Jaafar received a sentence of two years, with a non-parole period of eighteen months.

As for his two cohorts, during the course of the investigation a second weapon was located in the rear of a shopkeeper's yard, which was along the route that the third offender, Huang, had taken on foot. Among the many items he'd discarded during his getaway were a shoe and a white dust mask, both of which had DNA that matched with Huang's DNA profile. But in order to secure a conviction, Detective Beaumont had to return to the scene and locate a shopkeeper who'd witnessed a male running from the bank towards Coles' supermarket. His description of the offender matched that of Huang, and he further indicated that he saw the man remove a white dust mask as he ran. The last sighting of the offender was made within a short distance of where the dust mask and shoe were found. Huang was subsequently charged with aggravated robbery, depriving a person of their liberty, three counts of robbery in company and one count of robbery and assault. He received a sentence of five years, with a non-parole period of three years. He appealed his conviction, but it was dismissed.

To date there is still one offender at large. However, there is a fingerprint outstanding from the scene that has yet to be matched, along with numerous other unidentified prints from the exhibits that were examined.

6 The Body in the Wheelie Bin Murder

'No good deed goes unpunished.'
~ Clare Booth Luce

At around 10 pm on 29 June 2003, Redfern resident Charles Pryor decided to take out his garbage. It was a pleasant, cool evening in the Sydney suburb, so he was in no particular hurry. As he disposed of his trash he noticed a wheelie bin with an object sticking out of the top, almost directly opposite his house, on the corner of Renwick Street and James Street. Not being an area where wheelie bins were used, Pryor thought it was odd and went over to check it out. He extended his arm and probed around the object, which was covered up, and it felt soft. Instinctively, he knew it was a body. Alarmed, he hurried back indoors and called the police, who were on the scene within twenty minutes.

They extricated the body with care, discovering that it had been dumped head first into the bin with its feet protruding at an odd angle from the top. A blood stained Caribee sleeping bag with, in the circumstances, the rather ironic words 'Live the Adventure' printed on it covered the top half of the deceased down to the thighs and two black plastic garbage bags covered the legs. Police also found a box of cornflakes, a meat tray, a pair of shoes and, not surprisingly, a large amount of blood.

A crime scene was established, and the cadaver was duly taken to the Glebe morgue for a post-mortem examination. While that was going on, a number of constables spent the night looking for clues as to how the man had died, and when his body had been dumped in the wheelie bin.

The post-mortem, carried out by Doctor Paul Botterill of the Department of Forensic Medicine, Glebe, found that the cause of death was not completely clear and, although the findings were accentuated by the positioning of the body in the wheelie bin, the features were consistent with strangulation.

The toxicology report showed a blood morphine level of 0.2 milligrams per litre, as well as heroin (diacetylmorphine), monoacetylmorphine (a breakdown product of heroin) and acetylcodeine (an impurity which often occurs in street-grade heroin) in the stomach. Heroin rapidly breaks down into morphine in the body, and users or addicts generally inject it. However, because of where it was detected, the toxicology findings strongly suggested that the heroin had been consumed orally, which was most unusual. Morphine and codeine were also detected in the urine, indicating the deceased had been alive for some hours after consuming the drug.

As heroin was involved, it appeared prudent to eliminate the possibility of the victim being a drug user, so a sample of his hair was forwarded to the Victorian Institute of Forensic Medicine (VIFM) for analysis, hair being a useful sample to test because it can provide a drug history of the deceased. The results showed no detection of morphine or 6-monoacetylmorphine, only codeine. If the deceased had been a user of heroin, morphine and/or monoacetylmorphine would have been detected in the hair sample and, if he'd been a regular user, all three drugs would possibly have been found. Codeine is present in a wide variety of pharmaceutical preparations, including cough mixtures and various pain relief preparations, which contain paracetamol along with codeine. The deceased was clearly not a regular user of heroin, and the drug had most likely been placed surreptitiously in a drink, as the stomach contained some turbid fluid where heroin and its breakdown products were detected.

After extensive enquiries over several weeks, Redfern detectives identified the deceased as Shoukat Ali Mohammed, an Indian national, and they started tracing his recent history and movements. Further enquiries showed he was thirty-one years old and had arrived in Sydney from India in February 1998, on a student visa. He'd obtained casual work with a contract cleaning company, Baggett and Markham Services, and had last worked at the East Village Hotel on Palmer Street, Darlinghurst on the morning of 29 June 2003.

It also transpired that he'd met a fellow countryman, Deepak Singh, three years earlier in the Surry Hills area. Singh had previously travelled from India to Australia in 1999, and Mohammed had introduced Singh to the principals of Baggett and Markham Services, who subsequently employed him whenever Mohammed was unable to attend work.

Any acquaintances or friends were of interest to the police, and they discovered that during 2002 Singh had shared a Redfern residence with Youssef Tecle Imnetu, a Belgium national (also of Indian descent) who was better known as Joe but, in 2003, Joe moved into a two-bedroom home in Cleveland Street, Redfern, sharing with others. Deepak Singh was a regular visitor to the unit and, during that time, Shoukat Mohammed received a $178,000 settlement for a workplace injury. Several people were aware of the windfall, including Deepak Singh, who persuaded his friend to give him twenty thousand dollars to pay for a bridging visa after his student visa had expired.

Determined to leave no stone unturned, police examined CCTV footage from the Cleveland Street units for the day Mohammed was discovered. It showed him arriving at the units and parking his car in the underground car park at about 2.30 pm. Deepak Singh joined him, and together they left the car and entered the internal lift. Later, at 6.59 pm, the security camera recorded Deepak Singh leaving the car park lift and then the building through a security roller door that opened onto Renwick Lane.

A few moments later, he re-entered with a wheelie bin, which he took to the lift. At 8.15 pm both he and Joe Imnetu were recorded leaving the elevator. Singh was seen pushing the wheelie bin with something dark protruding from it. It was wrapped in black plastic. Joe Imnetu walked in front of him. Later,

Singh and Imnetu were again recorded on the security camera; this time getting into Shoukat Mohammed's car and driving it from the car park. Just under two hours later, Shoukat Ali Mohammed's lifeless body was found by Mr Pryor.

Joe Imnetu moved from Cleveland Street, Redfern around 6 July, 2003, while Deepak Singh left Australia on a Malaysian Airlines flight to New Delhi, India, on 17 July, having been deported for being in breach of his student visa. At the time, police had no idea of his involvement in the crime. But that was to change quickly because, just two days later, a search warrant was executed at the Cleveland Street address. Bloodstained carpet in the bedroom formerly occupied by Joe Imnetu was found along with a piece of bloodstained electrical cord, complete with switch. It appeared that Mohammed had most likely been murdered in the bedroom and that Joe Imnetu had spent the last week (after the murder), sleeping in the room before moving out.

Police inquiries revealed that Joe Imnetu had met with another person at Sydney Town Hall, where he'd apparently told them that some people had come into his unit, blindfolded him and told him to dispose of the body in the rubbish bin. Further investigations showed him to be very much a person of interest in the crime.

With evidence beginning to stack up against him, police 'invited' Joe for an interview. Realising it was a question of either going along with this 'voluntary' gesture or being arrested at his flat, Joe attended Redfern police station at about 6.20 pm on 1 August, breaking down and confessing to his participation in the murder.

Initially, he said that he couldn't remember what he was doing on 29 June, but later changed his mind, saying that Deepak Singh and Shoukat Ali Mohammed had in fact both been at the Cleveland Street apartment at about 2 pm that day. He'd gone out with Singh in the afternoon, leaving Mohammed alone in the unit. He further said that he'd left about 10 pm, returning about midnight before going to sleep. When questioned further, he denied having gone to the basement car park at any time on 29 June. However, the security footage clearly showed otherwise. His new address on Old South Head Road, Bondi Junction, was subsequently searched and a very incriminating black top with the insignia

DKNY on the front was found. The CCTV footage had shown him wearing it as Mohammed was being wheeled out in the wheelie bin.

On 14 June 2005 he stood trial in the NSW Supreme Court, accused of slaying Shoukat Ali Mohammed on 29 June 2003. Crown prosecutor Dan Howard, Senior Counsel, said that the two men – Joe Imnetu and his flatmate, Deepak Singh – had been observed on security video footage in their apartment building taking a wheelie bin with something protruding from it shortly after Shoukat Ali Mohammed was believed to have been murdered.

The results of the post-mortem were entered into evidence, and Dan Howard subsequently called on a number of people who knew the deceased to show that he had not been a drug user.

I was also called on to express my expert opinion, backing up and confirming what I'd previously said about the analysis of the deceased's hair confirming one way or another whether the victim had been a drug user, and in particular of heroin.

During the trial, it was also revealed that Mohammed had been struck over the head with a baseball bat before being strangled with an electrical cord and dumped into the wheelie bin when he failed to succumb to an oral dosage of heroin.

On 26 August, Joe Imnetu appeared for sentencing after the jury found him guilty of the murder of Shoukat Ali Mohammed. He was jailed for a minimum of twenty years.

Without a doubt, the prime motive for the murder had to be greed. When the orally ingested heroin hadn't seemed to be working on the victim, more drastic measures had been utilised, with a deadly outcome. It was a shocking pay-back to a friend and, if it hadn't been for an alert local resident checking out the wheelie bin with its grisly contents, the perpetrators may well have got away with premeditated murder.

As for Deepak Singh, thanks to advice and tip offs from the victim's relatives, he was apprehended in India and sent back to Australia to face trial, where he too was found guilty of murder and joined his accomplice in gaol.

7

Death of a Drug Dealer: The 'Ecstasy' and the Agony!

'There are only three sins – causing pain, causing fear and causing anguish. The rest is window dressing.'

~ Roger Caras

MDMA (3, 4 - Methylenedioxymethylamphetamine or ecstasy) is a very popular drug of abuse. After cannabis and amphetamines, it's the third most widely used illicit drug in Australia.

The early morning of 11 March 2003 was filled with unpleasant drizzle. David Hudson, aged forty-four and a known drug dealer, scowled and cursed the weather as he drove along Beach Road, Bateman's Bay. He had better things to do with his time than chase up debts. Sean Galgey owed him a thousand dollars and Hudson's patience had worn thin. It was time to make good on the outstanding sum. In the meantime, another of Hudson's customers, David Florit, was already with Galgey. He was brokering a repayment, also for a thousand dollars, for some Ecstasy tablets which was to be in the form of money and/or sexual favours from Galgey's girlfriend. The drug dealer's world dances to its own particular tune.

Soon after Hudson pulled in to Galgey's premises, a heated argument broke out between the three men regarding the debts. There appeared to be no room for compromise or negotiation. The dispute became loud and aggressive with threats being traded all round. At one stage, Hudson attempted to punch both Florit and Galgey, and on another occasion, he chased Galgey down the road. When Galgey returned, the row and fighting continued. At that point, Hudson removed his shirt and trousers, leaving him standing in just a pair of boxer shorts. The other two men looked at each other, wondering what on earth was going on. Then Hudson started to dance in a bellicose manner in the front yard of the property, all the time becoming louder and more belligerent.

'He's gone berserk!' Galgey exclaimed, whereupon a violent fight broke out between the three men.

Florit got Hudson in a headlock which was so severe that both parties fell to the ground.

'Knock him unconscious', Florit screamed.

Galgey proceeded to kick Hudson between the legs and around the stomach area while punching him repeatedly.

'Quick, get the baseball bat', a breathless Florit shouted.

Galgey ran into the house and retrieved the bat from the laundry.

Returning to where Hudson was being held by Florit, he hit the restrained man brutally with the weapon, a number of times. As Hudson floundered, Florit and Galgey bound his legs with a belt taken from the trousers he'd previously removed. Galgey then went back inside the house and returned with a bed sheet, which they used to further bind Hudson. Despite him being trussed and helpless, Galgey and Florit continued the beating until Hudson lapsed into unconsciousness.

The disturbance they'd caused hadn't gone unnoticed and Galgey's girlfriend, realising that matters were getting out of hand, phoned the police. Shortly after, Senior Constable Ken Cropper and Senior Constable O'Neill arrived at the scene and found Florit sitting on Hudson. It was raining heavily and both Florit and Hudson were soaked.

Florit, indicating Hudson, spoke to the policemen.

'He's crazy. Watch him. He's dangerous. He was trying to kill us. He's high on speed. He's the most wanted man in New South Wales.'

'Yeah, okay', Senior Constable Cropper replied. 'Now get off him.'

Taking note of what Florit had said, he started to handcuff Hudson, but quickly realised he was unconscious.

'Are you okay?' he asked.

There was no response and Cropper could see that Hudson's face was turning blue. He put the handcuffs away and began expired air resuscitation. Further police arrived and cardio-pulmonary resuscitation (CPR) was tried, continuing until an ambulance came to take Hudson to Bateman's Bay Hospital. Meanwhile Florit was wandering around the crime scene searching for something.

'Excuse me', he said to the policemen in general, 'I know you're busy, but could I borrow your torch? I've lost my wallet in the front yard somewhere'.

Senior Constable Garten snapped back, 'Your wallet isn't a priority at the moment. This guy's more important'.

'But it's got six hundred dollars in it.'

Garten then replied, 'We can't lend you the torch, the police are trying to save his life'.

That upset Florit, who became agitated. He took a few steps away before turning back. 'I hope he dies. He's a piece of shit.'

Yet more police materialised, including Detective Sergeant Ed Freeman and Detective Senior Constable Clayton. Freeman asked Galgey what had happened.

‘It was self- defence’, he replied. ‘We had to protect ourselves. Don’t worry about it, it’s all over drugs.’

As the rain continued to pour down, the area was covered by a tarpaulin to protect the crime scene. Florit and Galgey were taken off to Bateman’s Bay police station for questioning, while Hudson was transported to the local hospital. He was in a critical condition and, as his condition deteriorated further, he was later transferred to Canberra Hospital, where he died about midday the following day.

A post-mortem was conducted, and according to the ACT Government Analytical Laboratory report, blood samples taken from the body were found to contain the following:

- MDMA (3,4-methylenedioxymethylamphetamine) 0.68 milligrams per litre,
- methylamphetamine 0.14 milligrams per litre,
- citalopram (an anti-depressant drug) 0.16 milligrams per litre, and
- cannabis and its major metabolite (delta-9-THC acid) were also detected.

The high concentration of MDMA was well above the therapeutic range (0.1 – 0.35 mg/L) for the drug, and together with the elevated level of methylamphetamine was considered to be odd because by the time the samples were taken, it was eleven and a half hours after the altercation, when half of the drug should have been out of Hudson’s system.

In contrast, the citalopram found in his system was within the therapeutic range (0.048 –0.243 mg/L), while the cannabis indicated previous usage.

Taken superficially, the high levels of these amphetamines appeared to account for Hudson’s very aggressive behaviour and were possible contributing factors to his demise.

However, other results from the post-mortem told a different story. Hudson had received a very severe hiding from a variety of sources. He had bruising to his neck – apparently from the headlock – as well as numerous bruises to his upper torso, liver and kidney areas, groin and lower body. They were the result of not only the punching and kicking he'd been subjected to during the altercation, but also, more significantly, Galgey's very liberal use of the baseball bat. Twenty-five different injuries were identified on Hudson's corpse, the most serious of which were around his main organs. His liver and kidneys had been very badly damaged, with the right kidney faring worse than the left.

That gave a clue as to why the levels of MDMA and methylamphetamine were so abnormally high so many hours after the altercation. There are three mechanisms by which the body ultimately removes drugs from the areas where they have been active: metabolism, storage and elimination. The removal of drugs such as MDMA and methylamphetamine are mostly via the liver, kidneys and biliary system. If any of them is damaged, for whatever reason, their efficiency is greatly reduced. An inefficient or damaged renal secretory mechanism will result in the build-up of drugs in the blood to potentially toxic levels. Hudson's damaged liver and kidneys certainly fitted that scenario, and so may well have accounted for the elevated levels of MDMA and methylamphetamine.

I attended Bateman's Bay Court House for the initial hearing and gave evidence regarding the levels of drugs found in Hudson's blood. I was particularly concerned that a potentially toxic level of MDMA had been found in his blood after so many hours. For me, it just didn't add up.

In my experience, patients who had died of MDMA toxicity had had blood levels ranging from 0.110 to 1.26 milligrams per litre. Hudson's was 0.68 milligrams per litre, which was in the median of this range. I concluded that that 'anomaly' had to be due to his injuries, and in particular, the damage suffered by his vital metabolic and excretory organs – his liver and kidneys. Essentially, their ability to metabolise any drugs had been severely compromised. My final statement (in part) noted that the presence of 3, 4 methylenedioxymethylamphetamine (or MDMA) most likely contributed to his observed behaviour at the time of the incident.

And there the matter appeared to end. Was Hudson's death a result of the drugs he'd taken, or the beating he'd received? There was no conclusive verdict.

However, some years later, an appeal was lodged into the original outcome, and the matter resurfaced in the Nowra District Court. On the first day of the trial, the Department of Public Prosecutions no billed the matter without any witnesses giving evidence. The prosecutor didn't think they'd be able to prove the assault by Galgey and Florit caused the death of Hudson, their defence still being the same – the drugs in Hudson's system were responsible for his death, not the assault.

Consequently, both men walked free.

8
Up in Smoke

'Fire is a good servant but a fearsome master.'
~ Anon

Deaths by fire are mostly accidental, and suicide by this method is extremely rare. Self-immolation, also known as self-incineration, occurs when a person pours a flammable liquid – usually petrol (or gasoline) – onto themselves and sets it on fire. That has been known to occur in three victim categories: those with psychiatric problems, personal reasons or political motivations. However, when a fire is deliberately set the case may be classified as homicide. When a body is found in the debris of a fire, it's essential to discover whether it was alive at the time and died of asphyxiation, or whether it was already dead and the fire was started to conceal a murder. Samples of blood from the corpse are taken at post-mortem and, if they reveal the presence of carbon monoxide, it's almost certain that the victim was still breathing when the fire was started. The presence of soot particles in the airways and lungs is another positive indication.

The police in the Sydney suburb of Kellyville were enjoying a relatively peaceful start to Christmas Day, 2002. It was very much business as usual, but with a definite sprinkling of festive spirit in the air. However, that was all to change at 3.45 am when a call was received reporting the discovery of the body of an adult male lying prone in the footwell behind the front seats of a burnt-out Tarago van. The body, which had been extensively burnt, with some areas of skin visible in an unburnt condition on the front, was clothed in the remnants of a burnt white polo shirt and burnt black track pants. It was a grisly sight and about to get worse: when the van door was pulled open, the soles of the shoes on the corpse's feet ripped off on account of the fact that they and the metal had fused together.

On removal from the vehicle, the body bore a pugilistic posture with characteristically clenched boxer-like fists – typical of burn victims, as the muscles in their arms seize up as a consequence of the heat of the fire. The back of the corpse's body was burnt and its front was covered with soot, with areas of unburnt skin. A cherry-red fluid exuded from the mouth, which could have been due to a number of things, although carbon monoxide poisoning was thought to be the most likely cause.

A blood sample taken at post-mortem indicated the presence of delta-9-THC 0.008 milligrams per litre and delta-9-THC acid 0.016 milligrams per litre in addition to a blood alcohol level of 0.249 grams per decilitre (100 millilitres). Such a combination would have been sufficient to render the man into a very deep sleep, if not comatose, as cannabis exacerbates the effects of alcohol.

The carbon monoxide level of the corpse was found to be 63 per cent saturation. A blood saturation level of 50 to 60 per cent results in unconsciousness and coma with intermittent convulsions, but a blood saturation level of 60 to 70 per cent leads to a coma with intermittent convulsions, depressed heart action, respiratory depression and very likely death. The deceased's blood saturation level of carbon monoxide together with the alcohol level and cannabis present meant that, aside from the burns sustained, death was almost certainly caused by severe respiratory depression.

Other post-mortem findings noted the extensive burns (about 60 per cent) suffered by the deceased, while the pharynx, larynx, trachea and main bronchi all showed sooty deposits on the mucosal surfaces.

Quite clearly, the deceased was still very much alive when the vehicle caught fire, although most probably in a very deep sleep.

After sifting the evidence, it would appear that suicide could be ruled out, as could murder, given that the body was not burnt more extensively and there was no accelerant present. It was just a tragic avoidable death caused by too much merrymaking.

A probable scenario is that the man had been out celebrating at a Christmas Eve party, where he'd drunk large quantities of alcohol and, on returning to his vehicle, he'd sat inside and lit up a joint. Already in a mellow mood, he'd probably drifted off to sleep, allowing the lit joint to fall from his hand onto the flammable materials in the van. In his state of intoxication, he'd have been blissfully unaware of anything untoward and would have been in a deep slumber as the contents of the vehicle slowly combusted, releasing deadly carbon monoxide gas and soot into the cabin of the vehicle and his lungs. While asleep, this deadly combination of alcohol, cannabis and carbon monoxide had taken his life. Essentially, his breathing system had been in the process of shutting down, which had resulted in his death. The extensive burns to his body had just completed the deadly process.

9 Drink Spiking: A Two-man Crime Wave

'Each betrayal begins with trust.'
~ ***Phish***

Drink spiking isn't a new phenomenon. It's been going on ever since man first walked on the Earth, but it was undoubtedly popularised in twentieth century movies, television shows and books with the infamous Mickey Finn; a drink laced with chloral hydrate in order to incapacitate the drinker so that the villain of the piece could perpetrate their dastardly deeds.

Since then, a large number of drugs have been used for this insidious crime, including Rohypnol (flunitrazepam). This drug has featured so often in various drug-facilitated sexual assaults (DFSAs) that it's become known as the date-rape drug. The authorities [Therapeutic Goods Authority, in particular] have placed restrictions on the use of such drugs but, in spite of their good intentions, the anticonvulsant drug clonazepam slipped through the regulatory net, aiding the many predatory drink-spikers that are always on the prowl. Unfortunately, that drug has now been implicated in a number of DFSA cases, other than the one featured in this story, albeit not on the same scale.

Clonazepam (Rivotril, Paxam) is a benzodiazepine drug that has been used as an anticonvulsant to treat generalised epilepsy in adults and children as well as restless legs syndrome and acute mania. It's the 2-chloro analogue of nitrazepam, which is also a potent sedative and has been used as a substitute for flunitrazepam. Generally administered orally in doses of 1.5 to 20 milligrams, in the form of 0.5 – 2 milligram tablets, it can result in central nervous system depression, including impaired alertness, transient amnesia, memory impairment and somnolence (sleepiness) in non-tolerant people. Those effects are exacerbated if alcohol is also consumed, and while the fact that the drug doesn't change the colour or taste of the liquid consumed is a positive for those taking the drug under medical supervision, that very positive becomes a major negative when in the hands of those up to no good.

Chebli Djait and Adel Samadi were two such people. In October 2004 the Sydney pair, working under the aliases of Andy and Dylan, engaged in what they believed was the perfect plan to not only liberate the property of unsuspecting victims but also, in the instances where the victims were women, to engage in free, no-questions-asked sexual relations.

Over a six-day period, they preyed upon those they thought were the most vulnerable in true conman style, oozing charm and bonhomie as they befriended their victims by taking them for drinks, coffee or lunch at a series of venues such as the Three Wise Monkeys on George Street, the Shark Hotel on Liverpool Street, and the Pontoon Bar and the Opera Bar at Darling Harbour.

Using their geniality to keep their victims off guard, Andy or Dylan would always find a moment to spike their drinks via a tic-tac dispenser, and over the course of the six days, they drugged twelve different people, ten of whom were female tourists. In most instances, they managed to get their victims back to their hotel rooms, where they'd await the right moment before stealing cash, jewellery, credit cards or whatever else took their fancy, and in the case of two of the women, raping them, whilst sexually assaulting others. The victims were then left to come round in their own time, usually the following day, with no memory of what had happened. They would find their property was gone and, in the cases of the women, that they had been raped or sexually assaulted in some other way.

Complaints were made to the police, and after extensive enquiries by city detectives over several weeks, Chebli Djait and Adel Samadi were arrested. Djait was picked up in Kings Cross on 19 October, in possession of a prescription for the drug clonazepam, and Samadi was arrested the following day with two bottles of the same drug in his possession. One bottle contained more than eighty-five tablets of Rivotril, while the other was filled with a white liquid containing clonazepam.

Blood samples were taken from five of the victims, and they all tested positive for clonazepam, ranging from 0.015 to 0.030 milligrams per litre. To put that into perspective, the therapeutic level is 0.01 – 0.024 milligrams per litre. Two other victims only provided urine samples, in which clonazepam was also detected.

I attended Sydney Central Court, a fine heritage-listed sandstone building, for the initial hearing, and gave evidence regarding the levels of clonazepam found in some of the victims' blood samples. As none of the victims were mentioned as suffering from epilepsy, the levels of the drug found in their blood were one and a half to three times higher than the lower end of the therapeutic concentration. In layman's terms this means they were given a good deal more clonazepam than was necessary to achieve the villains' objectives.

A twenty-four-year-old Korean student described her harrowing ordeal to the court. She met Andy and Dylan at the Shark Hotel on 17 October, and after they introduced themselves, they bought three rounds of drinks. She had a Midori and pineapple juice, and while they were all talking, she lost her memory. She didn't remember leaving the bar, so must have been helped to her room, where a number of sexual assaults were carried out. When she awoke the following morning, she began to recall snatches of what had happened.

'My eyes were open, but I couldn't see properly', she said. 'I couldn't think properly. I couldn't resist. He took off my underwear.'

She also told the court that she'd spent most of the day in a drugged sleep, and during that time she'd been assaulted three times by Andy.

Another victim, a twenty-two-year-old Japanese tourist, said she didn't recall leaving the Three Wise Monkeys bar, but woke up the next morning in bed with a man she knew as Andy.

Ms Susan Alexander, Head of Regulatory Affairs at Roche, which markets Rivotril, gave evidence regarding the effects of clonazepam, stating that unlike Rohypnol (a member of the same drug family), which had been modified to contain a dye so as to warn of its presence in a drink, Rivotril had undergone no such treatment, presumably because, as she said, 'Prior to this case there had been no evidence that Rivotril was being used as a substance of abuse'.

I found that last point to be particularly interesting as, at the time, I had several cases on file in which clonazepam had in fact been used in such a manner on a number occasions in the past.

Witnesses were deemed to have given sufficient evidence against Andy and Dylan for the matter to go before the district court.

As the trial began in the Downing Centre District Court, presided over by Judge Robyn Tupman, the jury was told of the characteristic *modus operandi* of the attacks by Andy and Dylan.

The first victim to give evidence was Ms Tracey Vo, who described feeling hazy and very drunk, and unable to see straight, with parts of the evening blacking out. Fortunately for her, she'd been able to get to the safety of a friend's hotel room before passing out.

Other victims hadn't been so lucky. One, a male, had invited Andy and Dylan home with him for a glass of wine, only to wake up the next day to discover seventeen thousand dollars worth of property had been stolen. Dylan's DNA was found on a sock in the apartment and Andy's fingerprints were found on a door.

Yet another victim said she'd woken up on a mattress in Djait's unit, fully clothed. However, she'd found that she'd been unable to move her head or body, essentially being paralysed. Andy had then removed her clothes and had sex with her.

Andy also faced three charges of sexually assaulting the Korean tourist at his apartment, while Dylan stood accused of sexually assaulting a Swedish woman at a Kings Cross backpackers hostel. Semen found on her sheets matched his DNA.

Of Andy and Dylan's victims, four were Japanese, two Korean, one Swiss, one Swedish, one was from Perth, another from Adelaide and two from Sydney. A veritable cornucopia of nationalities.

Adel Samadi and Chebli Djait were found guilty of drugging, robbing and raping multiple victims and were sentenced to fifteen years behind bars, with a non-parole period of twelve years. In sentencing the pair, Judge Robyn Tupman not only condemned what she called the serious and potentially fatal practice of drink spiking, but also found it disturbing that a doctor (Dr Makram Girgis) had prescribed Samadi and Djait the drug in a joint consultation and apparently hadn't monitored their treatment. That led her to the conclusion that it was their ready access to the drug, in an apparently uncontrolled manner, which had made the commission of their offences so much easier.

For his part, Dr Girgis later told reporters he didn't recall a joint consultation, but that he couldn't say anymore, as the matter was in the hands of the police, the medical board and the HCCC (Health Care Complaints Commission), who confirmed that he was under investigation.

While the trial was unfolding, Cheryl Khoury, Djait's partner, took it upon herself to make about forty-six phone calls to two of the female witnesses, threatening them if they testified.

In one call, she said, 'In half an hour you're going to be killed. You're going to die. We are watching you from outside now'.

When one of the witnesses asked her why, Khoury replied, 'Because you sent the two guys to jail and you're going to court. If you think the police are gonna save you, they can't save you, believe me. You put somebody in jail, you gonna pay'.

In another conversation, Khoury said, 'You caused big trouble. I know where you live. I know where you work. I know everything about you'.

She was subsequently charged with two counts of threatening a person with intent to influence a witness. As she waited in the public gallery, prior to her sentencing, she collapsed dramatically to the floor, crying repeatedly, 'I'm having an anxiety attack! Get me some tablets!'

After being helped from the floor by relatives, she left the courtroom in tears. Nobody was quite sure whether she'd had a genuine attack or had engaged in an extraordinary bit of acting.

Just under two months later, she appeared before NSW District Court Judge Ronald Solomon and pleaded guilty to the two counts of threatening a person with intent to influence a witness. Her psychiatrist, Dr Monier Younan, gave evidence on her behalf, stating that his '… patient suffered from a complex psychiatric condition with a mixture of psychiatric disorders. These include obsessive compulsive disorder, chronic anxiety, post-traumatic stress and depression'.

Judge Solomon recognised that Cheryl Khoury's offences deserved a custodial sentence, but in consideration of Dr Younan's evidence, he said it would be 'cruel and inhumane to send her to gaol', further adding, 'If I sent this offender to full-time custody, I would be perpetrating a harsh and unnecessary punishment'.

He then handed down a twelve-month suspended gaol term for each offence and placed her on a two-year good behaviour bond.

Cheryl Khoury didn't know just how lucky she'd been, as the offence she committed usually carries a maximum penalty of ten years imprisonment.

In light of the two women who underwent mistreatment at the hands of Andy and Dylan and were then threatened, one can't help but wonder if justice really prevailed that day.

10 A Strange Bait Box Death

'Life is pleasant. Death is peaceful.
It's the transition that's troublesome'
~ ***Isaac Asimov***

Four hundred and seventy-eight kilometres south of Sydney, bordered by Nullica State Forest, the delightful fishing village and historic whaling town of Eden is the most southerly settlement in New South Wales. Due to the sparkling clear waters, the area is also known as the Sapphire Coast. Located between Nullica Bay to the south and Calle Bay, the northern reach of Twofold Bay, Eden is home to the main port and fishing fleet in Snug Cove.

It was in this charming setting that Robert Mitchell was employed as a fisherman on a forty-five-foot longline tuna fishing vessel known as the *Joanne-Glenn*. It was driven from a small single-sized cabin at the front of the craft. Just behind the driver's cabin was a winching wheel used for catching the fish, and on either side of the winching wheel was a bait box or tank, both of which were used to preserve the bait. They were flush up against the port (left) and starboard (right) sides of the vessel. Due to the very early starts, Mitchell often slept on board the vessel, which was moored alongside a larger vessel, the *Delamere*, at Commercial Wharf, Snug Cove.

Monday, 28 March 2011 had been a typical day of hard work and toil. Up at the crack of dawn for a mammoth day of longline fishing, Mitchell and his colleagues were feeling quite bushed when the *Joanne-Glenn* returned to port. It had been a good catch of tuna and the mood on board was buoyant, but now the crew were ready to hit the nearest bar and start relaxing.

As he cast his eyes around the beer garden, Mitchell saw a couple of young women he recognised, chatting together.

'Hey', he said to his mate Dale Ballagh. 'Check out those two chickie babes.'

'Let's invite them over', Ballagh replied with a wink.

The young women sat down at their table and they all started talking and drinking. After a while, Mitchell headed off to the bottle shop to purchase additional supplies to take back to the boat, and the two men asked the women if they'd care to join them. On receiving an affirmative response, they made their way towards where the *Joanne-Glenn* was moored, but instead of inviting the women on board that particular vessel, they took them onto the larger *Delamere*, no doubt trying to impress them.

More alcohol was consumed, and a plate, some cannabis and a pair of scissors were brought out, with the women being invited to participate in the smoking of the drug. The four of them were getting quite intoxicated but the young women, sensing that things were starting to get out of hand, decided to leave. After they left, Mitchell and Ballagh engaged in a friendly tussle, with Mitchell putting Ballagh in a headlock, saying, 'We've stuffed a great night, mate!'

'Alright, alright, you've made your point', Ballagh protested. 'Let me go.'

Mitchell released him and they left the *Delaware* to climb aboard the *Joanne-Glenn*. The ship was dark and a drunken Mitchell wandered off. Ballagh waited for him on deck, assuming he'd gone to the toilet. However, after about ten minutes he started thinking that his friend was taking a long time just for a leak, and decided to go and find him. He searched the vessel and then the wharf, but could find no trace. *Where the hell is he?* he thought. *He's got an early start again tomorrow*. Ballagh couldn't leave without Mitchell, so at about 10.45 pm he climbed back onto the ship for yet another search. It was then that he came across a grim sight: Mitchell's legs were protruding from a bait box well. In desperation, Ballagh tried to pull his friend out, but couldn't do it. 'Help!' he called out. 'Help!'

His cries attracted the attention of Leanne Bradbury, who woke her son, Jacob. She asked him, 'Can you hear that outside? Can you hear someone calling out for help?'

Jacob listened for a few seconds and agreed that he could, so he got out of bed, dressed and, along with his father David, got into his car and drove down to the fisherman co-operative jetty, because that was where they thought the calls for help were coming from. On arrival, they realised the calls were emanating from the main commercial wharf, so they got back into their vehicle and drove over, parking about thirty to forty metres back from the *Delamere*. They got out of the car and ran over to the boat, which was partially illuminated by the inside cabin lights, and Jacob jumped onto the deck from the wharf. Then he hopped onto the bow of the *Joanne-Glenn*, which was in total darkness. Following the sound of the voice calling for help, he quickly discovered Dale Ballagh standing near the two bait tanks. Neither had a lid on.

'Help! Come help me pull him out', Ballagh shouted. 'He's gone into the tank. Come and help me, come and help me.'

Jacob could see two feet sticking out of the water, so he grabbed one leg while Ballagh seized the other, and together they tried to pull Mitchell out. But he was too heavy and their efforts were in vain. Further assistance was needed.

Jacob called out to his father, 'Dad, quick, come and help'.

David Bradbury ran over to help the two other men pull the body out. It proved to be difficult even with the three of them because of Mitchell's weight and the narrowness of the hatch. Eventually, they managed to get him about half way out, whereupon David Bradbury reached over and grabbed him by the shirt, and then together they were able to pull the body clear of the tank. As they did, a plastic pack of tobacco and other debris floated to the top of the water in the bait box, making it appear that Mitchell had been preparing a smoke before he plunged in.

They laid Mitchell's body on the deck and Jacob rang 000, asking for an ambulance. Meanwhile, Ballagh carried out CPR, but when Jacob rolled the body over a quantity of water ominously poured out of Mitchell's mouth. Ballagh kept up the CPR until the ambulance arrived, giving way to the paramedics who tried unsuccessfully to revive Mitchell. The police were then called, and they examined the area and spoke to the three men before allowing the body to be transported to the local hospital, where Mitchell was formally pronounced dead.

At the post-mortem, a blood sample showed the following:

- delta-9- tetrahydrocannabinol (delta-9-THC) 0.005 milligrams per litre,
- delta-9-THC acid 0.013 milligrams per litre, and
- alcohol 0.285 grams per decilitre (100 millilitres) of blood, while a vitreous humour sample was found to have present alcohol 0.305 grams per decilitre (100 millilitres).

That was a useful toxicological sample. Let me explain why.

A man eliminates alcohol from his system at a rate of between 0.010 grams per 100 millilitres per hour to 0.025 grams per 100 millilitres per hour, with the most likely elimination rate for most individuals being about 0.015 grams per 100 millilitres per hour. The difference between the alcohol content in Robert Mitchell's vitreous humour and his blood sample indicated that he was in the elimination phase and that he was a regular drinker of alcohol.

People with a blood alcohol concentration of 0.285 grams in 100 millilitres or above are under the influence of alcohol to the extent that there is substantial impairment of their motor skills, and in particular, their emergency reaction skills. Cognitive, motor and visual functions such as reaction skills, tracking ability, motor co-ordination, perception, judgment and decision-making skills are substantially weakened at that blood alcohol level and above. Judgment of time and distance is also hindered by alcohol, and decision-making can be compromised as a result of altered perceptions and/or incorrect judgment. That can result in a person not recognising a dangerous situation and consequently suffering a reduction in the time available to take evasive action.

Delta-9-THC acid is the active metabolic product of tetrahydrocannabinol (delta-9-THC), which, in turn, is the major psychoactive drug present in cannabis. Delta-9-THC causes changes in memory, motor co-ordination, judgment and decision-making skills, cognition and sense of time. The regular use of cannabis results in slowly increasing concentrations of not just delta-9-THC, but also, more importantly, its metabolite delta-9-THC acid, which has a longer half-life than the parent compound. When inhaled, delta-9-THC is rapidly absorbed from the lungs into the blood stream, with peak blood concentrations being reached within eight minutes from the commencement of smoking. However, those peak blood levels decline rapidly, reducing to between 5 and 10 per cent of their original level within the first hour. The time required to distribute half of the administered dose of delta-9-THC from blood to fatty tissues (THC is a lipophilic drug) is about thirty minutes, and within about two hours of sampling, the level of delta-9-THC is reduced by approximately 90 per cent. The impairment caused by cannabis is also exacerbated when combined with alcohol, resulting in clumsiness, uncoordinated movements and significant unsteadiness, making a person more accident prone and more likely to trip or fall over.

Given all the above, I concluded that the level of alcohol together with presence of cannabis (in particular, delta-9-THC) in Robert Mitchell's blood would have substantially undermined his ability to save himself in any emergency situation which may have existed on the fishing vessel.

We'll probably never know exactly what happened to Robert Mitchell, but it's highly likely that he was either looking for a toilet, given the amount of alcohol he'd consumed, or he was attempting to prepare and light a cigarette, a theory supported by the pouch of tobacco found floating in the bait box. However, with his level of intoxication, exacerbated by cannabis, he would have been quite unsteady on his feet, and so most likely stumbled and accidentally fell into the bait box and drowned. The injuries sustained to his head and neck were consistent with a fall and struggle, which he would have engaged in in an attempt to save himself from drowning. If the lids had been securely placed on the bait tanks, he would probably have only suffered a few bruises and maybe a hangover.

Sadly, that was not outcome.

A subsequent inquest found that Mitchell's was an accidental death caused by an excessive consumption of alcohol and cannabis.

There is some debate as to whether bait boxes are even necessary. Longline fishing involves live fish being impaled on hooks as bait. Prior to that, the live fish need to be stored in bait boxes full of salt water. If fish offcuts or artificial baits/lures were used instead, the fish wouldn't have to endure the suffering they currently do and the bait boxes wouldn't be necessary, making accidents like the one that happened to Robert Mitchell impossible, and a twenty-nine-year old man would probably still be alive.

11

The Lady in the Bath Water

'Chains of habit are too light to be felt until they are too heavy to be broken.'

~ ***Warren Buffett***

Propofol (2, 6-diisopropylphenol) is a short-acting intravenous anaesthetic drug used as a preoperative treatment in hospitals. It's available under the trade name of Diprivan and is a sedative-hypnotic which is used as an intravenous anaesthetic agent. It's available as an oil/water emulsion in 20 – 100 mL vials that contain 10 mg/mL as the free acid.

Abuse of propofol appears to be rare, although it featured in the death of the American singer Michael Jackson on 25 June 2009. The Los Angeles County Coroner ruled that he'd suffered acute propofol intoxication, although a sedative (lorazepam or Ativan) was also a contributory factor.

Propofol's use is characterised by a quick onset of action, a short duration of activity, and a dose-dependent depth of sedation. That means the depth of anaesthesia can be induced according to the dosage given to the patient. It's well known that propofol administration – even as a therapeutic dose – can cause respiratory depression, so oxygen and respiratory assistance is generally needed, with its use being more appropriate in a hospital setting, where such facilities are available.

Propofol has gained a reputation of being a popular recreational drug, particularly amongst young health care professionals, who have ready access to it, because of the euphoria, sexual hallucinations and disinhibitions that have been observed with propofol anaesthesia. One female radiographer even described the preparation as 'the milk of human kindness' before the drug, ironically, took her life. And that's not the only recorded tragedy.

Doctor Linda Goodhart was a well-respected anaesthetist. She was very professional and highly regarded by her colleagues and assisting nurses. She'd recently passed her Fellowship in Anaesthetics and was on her way to becoming a consultant – the pinnacle of her career – and she was still only in her thirties. Linda was a social animal and had many friends in Sydney, although most were doctors and various other professionals. Despite her physical attractiveness, she led a troubled love life and her boyfriends treated her poorly. One in particular Dan, a regular visitor to her apartment, was into drugs and violence, and on one occasion he caused an injury to her face. She texted him later to say: 'My whole eye and cheekbone is bruised and I'm seeing double'. Her relationship with him appeared to be mainly based on sex and drugs (such as cannabis and cocaine). That Dan didn't value her as she deserved and treated her badly was obvious to all and sundry, and her friends urged her to get out of the relationship. But to further complicate things, Linda was having an affair with another doctor at the same time, which caused her a lot of emotional pain during their time together. The other doctor was in a de facto relationship and was even with Linda the weekend before he got married. What a tangled web we weave ...

Nevertheless, Dr Goodhart didn't allow the complications of her love life to interfere with her work, always performing her duties well, exhibiting great clinical skills and showing great empathy towards her patients. But on the morning of 18 June 2006, that was all to change.

She was rostered on as the emergency obstetric anaesthetic registrar, but failed to show. At first, it was assumed she'd been held up in traffic or by some other minor inconvenience, but as the morning wore on and she failed to respond to phone and page calls, her colleagues started to grow concerned.

At 10.30 am, the switchboard advised Dr Howard, another anaesthetic senior registrar, that she hadn't arrived at work for her 8 am start and inquired if he knew where she was. 'This is so out of character for her not to show up for work without calling', he said. He then attempted to call her on her mobile and landline without success, at which point the consultant anaesthetist asked him to go to her apartment to check everything was okay. He arrived at about 11 am, but was unable to gain entry, so he sought out the security manager for the apartments and expressed his concern for Linda's welfare. Understanding his anxiety, the manager phoned for a locksmith, who arrived at 11.45 am and succeeded in gaining entry to the modest one-bedroom apartment.

Apart from the bedroom, it contained a separate bathroom and an open area living room with a connecting kitchen and adjoining exterior balcony. As the three men entered, they passed bloodstains on the tiled floor outside the bathroom, near an unplugged television set. The bathroom door was ajar. They went in, hearts in mouths, and found Linda Goodhart's naked body lying in a foetal position, partially submerged, in the bath tub. Inserted in her arm was an intravenous cannula with a syringe attached, which was gently floating in the bath water. The locksmith immediately rang for the police and an ambulance.

When the police arrived, they established a crime scene and took brief statements from the three men. The CSI (crime scene investigation) team then examined the area and photographed various items.

On one corner of the bath there were four green candleholders, each containing a burnt-out candle, and there was black sooting on the tiles above. In a nearby waste bin, they located a black mobile phone and an empty vial of Diprivan. Wrappings and medical paraphernalia were found throughout the apartment, as were copious supplies of Diprivan.

The quantity of Diprivan found posed the question: Did she commit suicide or was it an accident caused by recreational use that had gone terribly wrong?

After her body had been conveyed by government contractors to the local hospital for death certification, police carried out a further inspection of the apartment, finding two more vials of Diprivan in a toiletries bag in her bedroom cupboard, along with two vibrators and numerous condoms. As propofol can be used to induce and enhance sexual pleasure, it suggested that the supplies were for recreational use and that Linda's death had been accidental.

A blood sample taken from Linda's body at the post-mortem was found to have present propofol 2.6 milligrams per litre. Her urine sample was found to have present 0.8 milligrams of propofol and her bile sample 3 milligrams per litre of propofol.

For the induction of anaesthesia, blood levels of between 6 – 10 milligrams per litre are necessary, but during maintenance of anaesthesia, levels of about 2 –4 mg/L are sufficient. The level of propofol found in Linda's blood was within this latter range, and the presence of modest levels of the drug in her urine and bile indicated she was alive for some time before she became immersed in the bath water. Therefore, it was concluded that assisted death or murder was unlikely. That reasoning was further backed up by the number of needle marks on her body, which suggested regular usage of the drug.

The risk of death due to self-administered propofol intoxication is low, mainly due to the low concentration found in commercial vials (20 ml containing 200 mg propofol or 500 mg/50 ml in a pre-filled syringe). That's equivalent to a standard dose of 2 – 2.5 mg/kg body weight for the induction of general anaesthesia. The fast-acting narcotic effect of propofol (one to two minutes after injection) prevents self-injection of more than one vial at a time. Linda Goodhart would have been well aware of that, although health care workers such as medical and nursing staff who have easier access to the drug, have a greater potential for addiction, and deaths have occurred through over dosage.

The number of vials of propofol found in Dr Goodhart's apartment gave rise to the reasonable assumption that she had used the drug regularly and enjoyed its effects, thereby developing some degree of tolerance. And given her stressed environment, it may well have been her only way of achieving some degree of emotional and sexual fulfilment.

On the night of her untimely death, it's very likely that she'd returned from a difficult hospital shift and was seeking some physical and mental relief. After some attempts at inserting the cannula (hence the blood stains in the hallway), she slipped out of her clothes and into a warm bath (having previously lit the candles for mood) to relax and enjoy the effects of the drug. It was probably something she'd done on many previous occasions with no problem, but, unfortunately, that night was going to be quite different. Her fatigue from work may have been worse than usual and, as she rested, she drifted off to sleep and her head slipped beneath the bath water. Blissfully unaware, she would have been asleep as she drowned.

In his report, the pathologist wrote: The presence of pulmonary oedema and generalised organ congestion is consistent with both administration of an overdose of a respiratory depressant agent and death due to immersion.

I opined that it would appear that the propofol was self-administered, probably recreationally, resulting in respiratory depression and consequent anoxia with the possibility of immersion, resulting in her death. I had to agree with the pathologist that death was due to immersion, essentially drowning. However, I also wrote: the level of propofol present in her blood, in an apparently tolerant person, does not appear to be excessive, though quite sufficient to result in central nervous system depression.

It's an unfortunate trait of humans to resort to substance abuse to relieve stress from overwork and/or poor relationships, sexual or otherwise. A subsequent inquest found that Linda Goodhart's was an accidental death with propofol a contributory factor in the snuffing out of a promising young medical professional's life, just like the flames of the candles found in her bathroom.

As Sir Elton John so eloquently put it in his song about the death of Marilyn Monroe, a young movie legend of comparable age: *'she lived her life like a candle in the wind...'*

And so it appeared, did the good doctor.

12

The 'Cheese Ball' Killer – The Car as a Murder Weapon

'Before you embark on a journey of revenge, dig two graves.'

~ Confucius, China's most famous Teacher, Philosopher and Political theorist (551 – 479 BC)

Eli Westlake was a very likeable young man. Twenty-one years old, a bit of a character and, by all accounts, a promising young musician. Music ran in the family, his father being composer Nigel Westlake. He was very close to his elder brother Joel, and they often socialised together. On Friday 6 June 2008, he went to his brother's home and joined him and a group of friends recording music and drinking. It was a regular event, as Eli was establishing himself as a DJ on the Kings Cross nightclub scene. When they left Joel's home shortly after 2.30 am, they went to St Leonard's Tavern to continue the party, emerging in high spirits an hour or so later. As they were all walking home, they went into a 7-Eleven convenience store, where Joel bought a pack of cheese and bacon balls. It was then 4 am.

Meanwhile, Sarah May Ward was also enjoying an evening out. She was with her companion William Long, having earlier also been with a couple of friends, Anthony Gilbert and Lisa Polombi. Her evening kicked off at Mr Gilbert's home in Artarmon, where Sarah smoked two cones of cannabis, consumed a bottle of wine and took four five-milligram tablets of Valium (her regular dose was two tablets per day). After that, the group went to visit friends at the Sebel apartments before decamping at around 11 pm to the nearby Monkey Bar at Chatswood. There, Sarah took an ecstasy tablet, which she washed down with a glass of wine. She and her friends then returned to Artarmon at about midnight and they all watched television until Anthony Gilbert and Lisa Polombi went to bed, leaving Sarah and William drinking.

Over the next couple of hours, Sarah put away another bottle of wine, and at about 4 am, she and William decided to drive Anthony Gilbert's Toyota Lexcen to St Leonard's to buy some cigarettes. Twenty minutes or so later, as they were parking outside the supermarket in Christie Lane, they encountered Eli and Joel Westlake, along with their two friends, Jesse Horn and Toby Finlayson. Eli was in a playful mood, and on seeing the couple in the vehicle, he reached into the bag of cheese balls and threw some of them into the air like confetti, shouting, 'Happy honeymoon!'

Some of the cheese balls landed on the car's bonnet and a few found their way into the vehicle. Sarah Ward was not impressed. She got out of the vehicle in a very aggressive and confrontational mood and tried to hit Eli's brother before trying to punch and kick Toby Finlayson, who responded by crying out, 'Settle down. It's just chips. What are you doing?'

The lads moved off, thinking that was the end of the incident, and sauntered down the alleyway, away from the vehicle.

In the meantime, Sarah Ward got back into the car. She was fuming and sat in the driver's seat muttering to herself, while William Long sat beside her in the passenger seat. After a while, she said, 'I've had enough of those guys'.

She then gunned the accelerator and drove the vehicle in an erratic manner onto Lithgow Street, where Eli Westlake and his friends were walking. Unfortunately for Eli, he stood out from his friends because he was wearing a white sloppy joe, which was easily picked out by the car headlights. Ward drove toward the group, hitting Eli on the legs as he tried to get out of the way.

'What did you do that for?' he cried out, limping away from the scene.

Meanwhile, a CCTV camera located outside the Cabana Bar was silently recording the unfolding scene. Toby Finlayson, realising things were getting out of hand, shouted out to his friends, 'Run, let's get out of here. This is crazy'.

The four of them took off and hid in fear behind the industrial skip bins in Lithgow Street, believing that they provided a temporary safe haven.

But Ward had other ideas. She reversed the vehicle and then turned off the lights, lying in wait. A predator waiting for its prey.

After a short time, the four friends, thinking the danger was over, emerged from their cover only to be greeted by a high beam flash of headlights. The car powered forward. As with the proverbial rabbit caught in the headlights, it was too late to run. The car drove over the kerb, crossing a grassed nature strip, and hit the leg of Jesse Horne, who went up over the bonnet and landed on the kerb, suffering bruising to the right side of his body and lacerations on his hands from the windscreen wipers.

Eli Westlake was not so lucky. He was knocked down by the impact and his body remained pinned under the car as it careered down a set of steps to the entrance of the Oxygen gymnasium at 67, Lithgow Street, coming to rest on the tiled floor at the bottom of the steps, with Eli's body still underneath.

William Long took to his heels, but Sarah Ward got out of the vehicle and stayed at the scene. Police and ambulance were called immediately, although at the time, no one realised Eli was under the assault vehicle.

Eli's brother was the one who discovered him pinned under the front of the vehicle at the bottom of the stairs, his presence being given away by an ever-widening pool of blood. He held the hand of his dying brother trying to comfort him. 'Please help', he pleaded, unable to contain his tears. 'My brother's been killed.'

Sarah, Toby and Jesse (in spite of his own injuries) joined Joel, and together they tried to lift the vehicle off the now deceased Eli, without success. When the police and ambulance officers arrived a short time later, Joel Westlake, now aware that his brother was dead, turned to one of the police officers and vented his anger and grief. 'That's my fucking brother. He's dead.' Then turning to point at a hysterical Sarah, he added, 'And that bitch killed him'.

Sarah was subjected to a breath test on an Alcolizer 11653, which recorded a positive reading of 0.196. She was immediately placed under arrest.

Several times she then asked Constable Glenn Hockley, the arresting police officer, 'Is he dead?' adding, 'I think I killed him'.

Hockley replied, 'I don't know. Just take a seat in the back (of the police car)'.

The usual formalities for such a tragic situation were carried out before Sarah Ward was taken to Chatswood police station for the purpose of a breath analysis, which returned a positive reading of 0.145 grams of alcohol per 100 millilitres of blood. Given the circumstances, it was also necessary to also get her to give a blood and urine sample, so she was taken to the Royal North Shore Hospital.

At 6.30 am, her blood sample was taken by Dr Earl Abraham and her urine sample by Nurse Wanda O'Grady. Given that the CCTV camera had recorded the event taking place at 4.28 am, the time of the blood and urine samples was important, as it made an accurate back calculation of Sarah Ward's degree of intoxication possible.

Later on that day, at 1.55 pm, the vehicle was removed by crane, revealing Eli Westlake's body in its entirety. He was lying on his right side with his legs bent up in front of his torso and his left arm stretched out in front of his body. There was an extensive amount of blood over his head and pooled around his body. It appeared to have come from his nose, mouth and right ear, indicating extensive cranial injuries. A quantity of the 'offending' cheese balls were found in the front seat of the motor vehicle.

About 2.05 pm, Eli Westlake's body was conveyed to the Royal North Shore Hospital, where a life extinct certificate was issued by Dr Jeremy Pallot. His body was then transported to the Glebe morgue for examination, to establish the extent of the injuries sustained in the incident which had resulted in his death.

In the meantime, Sarah Ward was in police custody, being questioned.

Today, the majority of police interviews are electronically recorded and include audio and video. This evidence can then be replayed, using the in-court display and sound reinforcement systems. At the time of writing, over one hundred and sixty courtrooms are ERISP (Electronically Recorded Interview of a Suspected Person) compliant. As you might imagine, defence lawyers aren't very happy about this, as they can't raise doubt that the police have in some way behaved inappropriately during the interview. Interviews, including the one carried out with Sarah Ward, which have been video-recorded also have the added benefit of permitting those in court to see for themselves the facial expressions and body language of the accused person.

Sarah Ward was interviewed on 7 June at Chatswood police station by Detective Senior Constable Matthew Harmer. After the usual protocols, explanation of rights and various other details including names of the participants and the age of the interviewee, the interview attempted to determine what had happened and the reasons why the incident had unfolded as it had.

Sarah Ward was asked to describe her evening up until the point where she and William Long had encountered Eli, his brother and their two friends, including details of how much and what she had had to drink. When she came to describe the confrontation, she alleged that Eli, Joel, Toby and Jesse had been very aggressive, hitting the car window and being verbally abusive towards her and William. She also said that there had been five of them, later referring to them as 'heaps of them'. Furthermore, she claimed that she had been physically assaulted by one of them.

She maintained that she had just been driving fast to get away from the scene, but that her companion had caused her to veer off the road and into the four friends because he'd grabbed the wheel. She seemed to be unaware that the fatal collision had taken place in another street and could offer no satisfactory explanation as to how the vehicle had ended up in Lithgow Street, although she did say that she'd tried to stop the car once it had hit Eli and Jesse.

After asking a few more questions about the incident, the police moved on to formalising the identification of the driver and passenger. It was clearly established that Sarah Ward had been the driver at the time of the offence and that she had never previously seen the four young men. By that time she started to get very emotional, possibly realising the enormity of the situation she was in.

Detective Senior Constable Harmer left briefly to get some tissues for her, while Detective Senior Constable Lawson continued the necessary formalities.

The interview was then suspended due to time constraints, with a further interview carried out by Detective Senior Constables, Matthew Harmer and Scott Lawson at 1.54 pm. In that interview, the footage from the CCTV camera was shown to Sarah Ward, with further pertinent questioning as they went through it in exhaustive detail.

She was then asked questions to find out more about her drinking history and whether she had taken any drugs and/or medication. That established her consumption of a number of drugs, including an ecstasy tablet and three cones of cannabis the previous day. She also admitted to having taken antidepressants and cocaine on other occasions as well as having a problem with alcohol, confessing that she was a binge drinker, often consuming two bottles of wine on her own in one session.

'How intoxicated would you be after that?' Detective Senior Constable Harmer asked. 'Sometimes I can handle it and sometimes I can't.'

'What happens to you when you can't?'

'I suppose I can get emotional and fight', came the reply. 'I've done it all, but not recently.'

The interview was concluded at that point.

Eli Westlake's post-mortem was carried out by Dr Rianie Janse Van Vuuren at 9 am on 8 June. It showed 'multiple bruises and abrasions to the body, both on the anterior and posterior surfaces. There was an almost linear abrasion to the head and the left posterior aspect of the head appeared deformed. There were petechial haemorrhages in the eyes and on the right arm, probably position dependent. The right hand had a washerwomen's appearance, which could be related to the post-mortem position. The mandible had a fracture of the right lateral aspect.'

Eli's body had clearly been badly damaged when the car impacted with him the second time. But more important were the severe head injuries he sustained in the onslaught. Those head injuries were itemised as follows:

- Base of skull fractures extending into temporal bones on both sides,
- Subarachnoid haemorrhages on brain,
- Cerebral swelling with parahippocampal gyrus herniation,
- Laceration to left uncus,
- Left optic nerve laceration,
- Multiple haemorrhages in floor of fourth ventricle and in pons.
- An x-ray revealed the extent of the injuries sustained by Eli when the vehicle smashed into him. Death was through extensive skull fractures and loss of blood.

A toxicological examination showed he had 0.186 g/100 ml of alcohol in his blood (preserved) - a high level, with a higher level in the vitreous humour (preserved) at 0.219 g/100 ml, and an even higher level in his urine (0.242 g/100 ml), which would suggest that the alcohol metabolism was in the excretory phase at the time of the slaying. No other drugs were detected.

The high alcohol content in his blood indicated that he was well and truly intoxicated, and that may have accounted for his playful, if not boisterous, behaviour when he threw the cheese balls onto the vehicle driven by Sarah Ward.

On 6 July, 2009, Sarah Ward appeared at a committal hearing at Sydney's Central Local Court in front of Magistrate David Armati, where she was accused of murder or, on alternative counts, aggravated dangerous driving occasioning death or dangerous driving occasioning death.

On behalf of the Director of Public Prosecutions, Ms Sally Traynor outlined the events of the night of 6 June, 2008.

A number of witnesses, including myself, came forward and gave evidence in relation to this matter. I was amongst the last to give evidence, and was there to interpret the levels of drugs and alcohol detected in Sarah Ward's blood samples and so determine how much she would have been affected at the time of the incident. The analyst's reports (carried out by the Division of Analytical Laboratories, Lidcombe, New South Wales) showed that at 6.30 am on 7 June, 2008, she had the following levels of drugs and alcohol in her blood:

- 3, 4-methylenedioxymethylamphetamine (ecstasy) 0.07 milligrams per litre,
- delta-9-tetrahydrocannabinol (delta-9-THC) 0.005 milligrams per litre,
- delta-9-THC acid 0.023 milligrams per litre,
- diazepam 0.22 milligrams per litre and it's metabolites: nordiazepam 0.07 milligrams per litre and temazepam <0.01 milligrams per litre along with venlafaxine <0.1 milligrams per litre, and more importantly
- alcohol 0.140 grams per decilitre (or 0.140 per cent) of blood.

While the level of cannabis was significant, along with the presence of diazepam (and its respective active metabolites), the major player was alcohol. I estimated that the level of alcohol in Sarah Ward's blood at the time of the incident was most likely 0.171 per cent, concluding that she was under the combined influence of alcohol and cannabis, with probable additive effects from diazepam, to the extent that her driving ability would have been substantially impaired. My prognosis was confirmed by another expert involved in this matter, Dr Graham Starmer of Sydney University, who considered that Sarah Ward's most likely blood alcohol concentration at the time of the collision would have been 0.176 g/100 ml (range 0.166 – 0.197 g/100 ml).

However, the most damning evidence was to come from the CCTV footage and, having viewed that, it was decided that there were more than sufficient grounds for the matter to go to trial.

On 23 November 2009, Sarah May Ward stood trial in the NSW Supreme Court at Taylor Square, Darlinghurst before Justice Roderick Howie for the murder Eli Westlake on the morning of 7 July 2008.

She pleaded not guilty, but the Crown wouldn't accept her guilty plea to the lesser charge of manslaughter.

Prosecutor Elizabeth Wilkins, Senior Counsel, said Sarah Ward had used her car as a weapon when she drove onto the footpath in pursuit of Eli Westlake and that CCTV footage of the incident showed it to have been a deliberate, controlled and predatory act.

Sarah's barrister, Mr Eugene Wasilenia, said his client had never intended to kill or seriously injure Eli Westlake, noting that her blood alcohol reading had been 0.171 at the time of the incident, more than three times the legal limit, and that she'd also had drugs in her system. He further contended that she'd been attacked earlier by some of Eli Westlake's friends, she'd been unfamiliar with the borrowed car and she'd been trying to get away from the scene. He also said that she'd had trouble reversing the car and had hit the accelerator in panic, as her passenger (Mr Long) had pulled the steering wheel to get the car under control before it had hit Eli Westlake.

However, Ms Wilkins said Sarah had aimed the car at the pedestrian in the white sloppy joe twice, reversing and trying again after Eli Westlake had jumped out of the way after the first attempt. She stated that the Crown's case was that the accused, on both occasions, had driven her motor car up onto the footpath in order to hit him, and that as the group had walked off, Sarah Ward had actually been following, stalking the boys in her car, driving down a one-way street the wrong way. It was a case where actions spoke louder than words. Turning to the jury, Ms Wilkins said, 'When you watch the CCTV, you will be satisfied this was a deliberate, controlled and predatory act by the accused. She was using her car as a weapon.

'She was out seeking revenge for what she perceived was the humiliation she'd suffered in the laneway.'

A number of other issues were also raised during the trial, including Sarah Ward's drug usage, her depression, her bipolar disorder and her possible psychological condition. But a crown witness, forensic psychiatrist Dr Allnutt, said she should still have been able to control herself, as she'd displayed no evidence of mania at the time of the incident.

The defence barrister, Mr Eugene Wasilenia, put it to the court that the incident should be considered to be a chance encounter and an instantaneous reaction to a series of events, and not a premeditated attack on Eli Westlake because of all the young men present that night he had not been the most deserving or worthy of Sarah Ward's anger.

That last comment, combined with the stress of the proceedings, proved to be too much for Eli's father, Nigel Westlake, who stood up and stormed out of the courtroom. A short while later, he was followed by Joel, who swore at Mr Wasilenia.

Justice Howie told the remaining members of the Westlake family to talk to the pair and remind them Sarah Ward was entitled to a defence. On that note, he adjourned the hearing.

After a trial of nearly four weeks, on the second day of deliberations, the NSW Supreme Court jury, by a majority verdict, found Sarah Ward guilty of murdering Eli Westlake. Sarah sat in the dock sobbing.

Justice Howie commented that Sarah Ward had been the aggressor by using her car as a weapon and that none of the young men had in any way been responsible for Eli Westlake's death. He added that it had been Sarah Ward's intention to cause serious harm to Eli Westlake in order to teach him a lesson, but she had not intended to kill him. He also noted that by trying to help Eli Westlake's brother and friends lift the car off him, she had shown some remorse, and so he accepted that she had almost immediately regretted her actions.

Notwithstanding that, he sentenced her to a maximum of twenty-five years gaol, and with time in custody, she will be eligible for parole in March 2027.

However, the sentence handed down proved to be no comfort for the Westlake family. Outside court, Eli Westlake's father made the following statement of his family:

> We have been sentenced to a lifetime of anguish. She set upon our boys and their friends and she didn't let up until she'd killed Eli. No courtroom can bring back Eli, no sentence can relieve the pain of our loss. The notion of justice has very little meaning for us because the worst has already happened. Eli is taken and nothing will bring him back. We struggle each day to come to terms with this fact.
>
> 'We've heard all the evidence, seen the CCTV footage of the night in question and we concur with the findings of the jury, as tragic as this is not only for us but for the family of the accused and the accused herself.
>
> He concluded that:
>
> The Crown revealed that Eli's life was taken by a complete stranger in a savage act of brutal violence. An act laden with evil intent. An act that can only be described as disturbingly predatory in nature.

13

Dr Suresh Nair - Cocaine Killer

'Drug misuse is not a disease, it is a decision, like the decision to step out in front of a moving car - you would call that not a disease, but an error of judgment.'

~ ***Phillip K Dick.***

When Suresh Surendranath Nair was ten, his Indian parents migrated from Malaysia to Australia. A decade later, they returned home, leaving Suresh to pursue a medical degree at the University of Sydney. His fellow students thought him a very polite and quiet student, yet he possessed a grubby sense of humour and a liking for pornography, which gave rise to some pointed comments beside his yearbook photograph under the title 'good points'. For example, one read: 'Well, he has a good sense of humour, albeit disgusting. When you think of Suresh Nair, you almost immediately think of grunting and unintelligible mumbling; primeval noises'. Another was: 'Give him a good Penthouse and he's happy', while one classmate even predicted that by 2011 he would be: 'Deregistered and exiled to the rainforests of the Amazon to live with cannibals'.

Suresh was never an outstanding student, but even so, he was able to make the necessary grades in medical school before completing his residency and embarking on surgical training, specialising in neurosurgery. The postgraduate component involved very long hours as an intern, with life and death decisions to be made on patients. For the most part, Suresh appeared to be a competent doctor and successfully completed his training requirements.

During his postgraduate training, he started to exhibit a weakness for drugs, cocaine in particular. A prominent brain surgeon and friend, Dr Charles Teo, defended him by saying, 'Suresh doesn't have a balanced life, no social life. He's very awkward with girls and in my opinion it seems like he can't relate to women'.

However, due to his strange behaviour towards his patients and evidence of drug usage, Dr Nair was suspended in 2004, and again in 2008, after which he was forced to undergo regular urine tests and work under supervision. Clearly, cocaine and/or substance abuse was playing an important part in his life. The second suspension related to his clinical practice, but there were more serious problems. Dr Patrick Cregan, a general surgeon and head of quality assurance at Nepean Hospital, told the Health Care Complaints Commission (HCCC), 'There are significant holes in the concept of supervised practice. It's a myth that you can supervise someone doing surgery'.

Such indecision, without any other firm guidelines, led to further serious problems, and Dr Nair continued to practice surgery while under the influence of cocaine and, possibly, other stimulants. Despite staff concerns, he was allowed to work under supervision at Nepean Hospital, a decision which led to unfortunate untoward consequences, resulting in a number of botched operations and, ultimately, the deaths of two young women.

We'll probably never know how many operations Dr Nair presided over from 2004 onwards that may have been less than adequate. That's something only his colleagues would be able to estimate. However, that's unlikely to happen given the focus of maintaining a doctor in practice where possible and delaying any necessary disciplinary measures. What we do know is that there appears to be a long list of patients who will never recover from what was done to them. Amongst those, two stand out, namely Ms Helen Kerner and Mrs Debbie Burns.

Helen Kerner trusted her 'nice, clean-cut' neurosurgeon when he said he'd performed the delicate spinal operation she required many times before. But when she woke up incontinent and still in pain, with no feeling in her legs or pelvis, she began to have second thoughts. And when he tried to discharge her from hospital two days into recovery, she became very upset. But the kicker came when Dr Nair confessed that his drill had slipped during the procedure, severing several nerves in her spine. Despite that, Helen Kerner said she felt sorry for the doctor, who was then 38. 'I felt like, "my goodness me, he must be feeling awful for what he's done". But not now. I'm pretty angry now.' Another neurosurgeon described the procedure, performed in 2006, as a standard operation and said Dr Nair's blunder was 'usually so rare as to be virtually unheard of'.

Helen Kerner, a former relief manager at Anglicare second-hand shops, said she didn't know Dr Nair had been suspended back in 2004 when she was referred to him in 2006. 'I had very bad back pain, sciatic pain, and all the doctor had to do was remove a bone spur away from the nerve, just grind it away from the nerve. The drill slipped, and my life changed, completely changed.'

She used to be a keen gardener and enjoy dancing, but now she has to use walking sticks because she can't feel her left leg and her foot is deformed. She's also bladder and bowel incontinent, lives with constant, severe pain in her legs and feet and has lost her sexual function. 'I'm very depressed', she said. 'I wake up in the morning crying sometimes. I'm very embarrassed to go out because of things that happen. That's my life now. I don't have one.'

She said she knew something was wrong when she woke from the anaesthesia. 'I spoke to Dr Nair the next morning and he didn't tell me he'd slipped with the drill. He said he'd stretched one of the nerves and it had to be repaired. He said within three months it should heal itself, and I believed him because he's my doctor.'

Her distress was further compounded when Dr Nair tried to have her discharged from hospital two days after the procedure, before she had been seen by a continence adviser and/or physiotherapist. It was not until Helen Kerner noticed the word 'severed' written on her observation chart that she sought answers as to her predicament.

Dr Nair only confessed his blunder when confronted at a meeting attended by the hospital's nursing manager, the hospital's clinical liaison officer, Helen Kerner and her partner at the time. After yet another meeting, Helen Kerner was advised by a friend, a continence advisor and two hospital administrators that she could sue for negligence. Legal proceedings began in November 2008 and Sydney West Area Health Services admitted to her solicitor to a breach of duty of care. The NSW Supreme Court is going to determine what compensation and damages NSW Health must pay.

Another botched operation concerned Mrs Debbie Burns.

Dr Nair operated on Mrs Burns – a forty-nine-year-old mother from Werrington – at Nepean Private Hospital, on her neck for spinal surgery on 29 October, 2010. The surgery left her unable to hold her head up. Mrs Burns said, 'I would do anything to go back to before. The pain that I was experiencing was far worse than the pain I had before the operation'.

She explained that when she woke up from her surgery she was in extreme pain, with no feeling in her left hand. Dr Nair assured her everything was normal and put her on morphine, saying she should stay in hospital until the following Monday. However, he telephoned her two days later and said he was too unwell to see her and that she could go home. Mrs Burns said she was then discharged with no pain relief medication and woke up the following morning in terrible pain.

'On the Sunday when I got out of bed, it was just terrible. I would stand up for five minutes and have to sit down for twenty minutes to rest my head', she said. 'It was excruciating pain. It felt like my head was too heavy for my body.'

On 11 November 2010, she was admitted to hospital for pain management after her husband, John, had complained to Dr Nair's secretary. The family then decided to get a second opinion and found out soon afterwards that Dr

Nair had been suspended in 2004. Further surgery was clearly necessary to correct the problem. However, Mrs Burns was told by her new surgeon that she may never regain feeling in her left hand. The Burns' family have since filed formal complaints about Mrs Burns' care with the NSW Medical Board and the Health Care Complaints Commission.

What Helen Kerner and Debbie Burns didn't know about Dr Nair was that he was a cocaine addict, charging thousands of dollars per operation to support his habit. It was the dark secret of a depraved life of cocaine, call girls and all night orgies.

Dr Nair was indulging himself in a way of life that most people can only dream about. His career as a successful neurosurgeon allowed him the financial freedom to host weekend parties that would rival any rock star's lifestyle.

In some ways, Dr Nair was indeed a rock star, only the 'rock' was a potent form of cocaine that he inserted into the bodies of young escorts who came to his luxury $1.7 million Elizabeth Bay apartment in the eastern suburbs of Sydney.

Life outside work was a party, and Dr Nair, now in his forties, had the money to pay for it. He also had a penchant for lovely looking model-type girls and desired sex under the influence of drugs, in particular, cocaine. He sought high-price escorts to satisfy his needs, and consequently, a stream of young women found their way to his sumptuous apartment.

A number of the young women came from HM Escorts, Sydney, and the financial rewards on offer made Dr Nair a very popular client. They would often arrive at his front door to be greeted by him offering lines of cocaine on a plate. He'd then urge them to remove their clothes and snort the cocaine before the bacchanalian activities began. Those cocaine and sex binges often lasted well into the morning, and as a consequence, they began to impact upon Dr Nair's duties as a surgeon and the lives of a number of people associated with him. However, when two of the girls died, his secret depraved life started to unravel.

The first of the girls to die was Victoria McIntyre, a pretty twenty-three-year old escort who attended one of Dr Nair's fateful cocaine sex parties. She worked part-time under the pseudonym of Lisa for HM Escorts and visited Dr Nair's residence on 15 February 2009. She was fairly new to the game and used the activities to supplement her regular, more conventional occupation in recruitment management.

By the time she arrived at the apartment, at 11 am, drug use and sexual activity were well under way, although one escort had left earlier when she refused to take the drugs. As she entered, Dr Nair told Victoria to get naked and take cocaine, although one of the other two escorts who were there, Elizabeth Carlson, told her, 'Be wary of the drugs being forced upon you'.

Victoria replied that the only reason she was there was for the money, and she failed to heed the warning.

Dr Nair then told the other two escorts, Juliette Lancaster and Elizabeth Carlsen, to leave the apartment to go and buy some sex toys. He also wrote out a prescription for Xanax before handing them some money. Juliette and Elizabeth then left the apartment and walked to Kings Cross to carry out their errands.

A short time later, Victoria began to suffer seizures, apparently from the excessive cocaine ingestion. Dr Nair attempted to provide medical support, but realised he was unable to help her and so called for an ambulance via the 000 service. In the meantime, Juliette and Elizabeth returned to the apartment with their purchases, minus the Xanax, only to be told by Dr Nair to come back thirty minutes later.

They both took a taxi to the Sydney Swans AFL club on Darlinghurst Road, Kings Cross and had a drink.

When the ambulance arrived a short time later, the ambulance officers were so concerned that Victoria would die that they contacted the police. She was quickly transported to St Vincent's Hospital where she was intubated and, on examination, emergency staff found her to be brain dead. She was immediately placed on life support in the Intensive Care Unit, and at 12.01 am, Monday, 16 February 2009, it became quite apparent no recovery was possible, and she passed away with family and friends present.

Strangely, Dr Nair, who had previously been suspended in 2004 and 2008, was not required to inform the NSW Medical Board of this woman's death in his apartment.

The second death involving Dr Nair was that of an attractive young escort by the name of Suellen Domingues-Zaupa. She hailed from Brazil and was a twenty-two-year old student. Fond of a good time, the fun-loving young woman had her philosophy expressed on her Facebook page: Life looks after those that live it. She also had a tattoo on her foot that read: 'The world is full of magic'.

She worked part-time for HM Escorts under the pseudonym of Nicky and was booked to visit Dr Nair's residence on 19 November 2009.

Like Victoria McIntyre, she was also new to the game, and she used her extracurricular activities to supplement her studies in hospitality management and travel around Australia. However, she must have been very discreet, as a flatmate later commented, 'The lifestyle she lived was by no means that of a high-class escort and none of us who knew her well believed she would be capable of doing such a thing'.

On the afternoon of 19 November, Colombian-born escort, Carmen Hernandez-Cardona spent four hours at Dr Nair's apartment, receiving a cheque of three thousand, two hundred dollars in lieu of services rendered. She then snorted half a line of cocaine with a fifty-dollar note.

Suellen arrived a short time later and was also given a cheque. She undressed and, after some kissing and cuddling, snorted some cocaine and joined Dr Nair and Carmen in a threesome sex binge that lasted close on four hours. As she was about to leave, Dr Nair gave her a further cheque to stay on, but then she began to shake uncontrollably, all the time having trouble breathing and talking in a crazy way, saying things like, 'I got bananas in my eyes'.

After about fifteen minutes, her face started to go a grey-blue in colour and bloody saliva began to emerge from her mouth. It was a sign that her bodily functions were shutting down.

‘Please, do something’, Carmen pleaded to Dr Nair.

‘She’ll be alright’, he replied. ‘I’m a doctor. Trust me.’

A short while later it became apparent that Suellen was dead, and Dr Nair offered Carmen fifty thousand dollars to keep quiet about what had happened. She refused the offer and left the apartment.

Meanwhile, back at Nepean Hospital, staff were growing worried that Dr Nair had been absent from his duties, with no explanation, for the past two days. Unable to contact him, they contacted the police at Kings Cross, expressing their concerns, and at about 7.30 pm on 20 November, a police patrol car was sent to his address in Elizabeth Bay.

Nobody appeared to be home, so they left a business card under the door requesting Dr Nair to contact them. No reply was received, and at so at around 2.30 pm on Saturday, 21 November, police returned to the premises and tried again. Once more, they were unable to gain access. Thinking something out of the ordinary must have happened, they forced an entry. When they looked in the main bedroom, they found Suellen lying face up on the bed. She’d been covered with a quilt, with a towel and two pillows placed over her head, and her legs were exposed beyond the quilt, showing that she was only wearing underpants. It was clear she’d been dead for some time.

Detectives and crime scene officers were immediately notified.

Officers examining the crime scene observed that the deceased had froth in her mouth and was clutching a new condom, removed from a packet, in her left hand. There were numerous other condoms strewn around the apartment, both opened and unopened, used and unused. Further searching revealed numerous glasses and empty bottles of vodka, together with abundant quantities of white powder.

It was later learned that several other escorts had been entertained in the apartment while Suellen’s lifeless body had lain on the bed.

Dr Nair was tracked down and on 25 November he was charged with supplying drugs in relation to her death. He was also immediately suspended by the NSW Medical Board for the third time.

Samples taken from Victoria McIntyre at the post-mortem showed her blood contained toxic levels of cocaine – 7.1 milligrams per litre – and its metabolite benzoylecgonine – 7.0 milligrams per litre. Cocaine was also detected in her nasal and rectal swabs while her post-mortem examination, in part, showed a focal haemorrhagic area in the heart. The lungs were congested and oedematous (filled with fluid). There were minor injuries to the anal and rectal area and some contusions in the bladder and an abrasion in the rectum. She clearly had a rough night.

Forensic pathologist Dr R Janse Van Vuuren concluded that in light of the fact that there was acute haemorrhage in the heart and focal haemorrhage in the brain in conjunction with high cocaine levels, the cause of death was acute cocaine toxicity.

The conclusion I reached in my final opinion was similar. I wrote that the extremely high level of cocaine detected in Victoria McIntyre's blood would have most certainly lead to her death.

The blood preserved sample for Suellen Domingues-Zaupa showed the following results:

- benzoylecgonine 3.4 milligrams per litre,
- cocaine: 4.9 milligrams per litre [Cocaine concentrations in fatalities range from 0.9- 21 mg/L (average 5.3 mg/L)],
- alprazolam (Xanax): 0.009 milligrams per litre [In seven cases of apparent suicide of adults by alprazolam ingestion, the post mortem blood concentration was 122 – 2100 ug/L (average 550 ug/L). The concentration of alprazolam detected in the blood of the deceased was therefore well below the toxic levels.],
- lignocaine: 2 milligrams per litre, and
- delta-9-tetrahydrocannabinol acid (an inactive metabolite of cannabis) 0.017 milligrams per litre.

Cocaine, levamisole and lignocaine (the latter two drugs are used as cutting agents for cocaine) were detected in her nasal and rectal swabs.

The post-mortem examination carried out by Dr Isabella G Brouwer showed that Ms Domingues-Zaupa's body was in an early state of decomposition. The internal organs were decomposing and had an autolytic appearance. Both lungs had a mottled appearance. She had clearly been dead for some time.

I also concluded in my report that the extremely high level of cocaine detected in Suellen's blood would have most certainly led to her death, although I was unable to comment on the level of levamisole, as the drug was not quantified. However, the ingestion of levamisole is potentially dangerous and should only be administered under medical supervision.

That appeared to be in agreement with the pathologist's reports and other expert statements. Both victims had died through the excessive ingestion of cocaine.

Suresh Nair was eventually charged with two offences: the murder of Brazilian student and escort, Suellen Domingues-Zaupa in November 2009, after she'd been supplied with a prohibited drug (cocaine) at his Elizabeth Bay apartment, and the manslaughter of fellow escort, Victoria McIntyre in February, 2009, again after she'd been supplied with a prohibited drug (cocaine). Incredibly, he was granted bail provided he didn't hire any sex workers or take prohibited drugs.

However, rather than thank his lucky stars that the Australian justice system was being ludicrously overgenerous and excessively fair (following in the footsteps of the NSW Medical Board), Nair continued in his ways. But unknown to him, he was placed under surveillance, and on 8 January, 2010, he was seen separately hiring three female escorts between 9.30 pm and 11.15 pm and taking them back to his first floor apartment in Hall Street, Bondi, where he partook in cocaine with two of them.

Police raided his apartment shortly after midnight. When the arresting officers knocked on his door, he answered and called out to the women in the bedroom, 'Girls, put your clothes on. The police are here. It's over'.

The police raid on the apartment came a week after Dr Nair had discharged himself from a private hospital, where he'd been undergoing treatment for his addictions as part of his bail conditions.

The extraordinary leniency previously granted to him was about to end.

In applying for further bail on 11 January, Dr Nair's solicitor, Mitchell Cavanagh, admitted to Sydney's Central Local Court that his client had a problem. He told the court that his client would not reoffend if he was allowed to live with his mother, and that he would stay at a psychiatric hospital if necessary. He added, 'He realises now he cannot trust himself to be on his own'.

The application was refused by Magistrate Jane Culver, who said, 'This is a matter where the protection of the community looms large. This court can have little confidence in the defendant's willingness to comply with bail conditions'.

Nair was taken into custody and transported to Silverwater gaol.

While in gaol, he was assaulted by four inmates, suffering multiple facial fractures, including a broken jaw and broken teeth. Because of the attack, he lost partial sight in one eye and was left without feeling in his left cheekbone. He was briefly placed in protective custody after the incident.

In a Supreme Court bail hearing on 25 June, 2010, his barrister, Peter Hamill, Senior Counsel, called on psychiatrist Dr Rosalie Wilcox to give evidence about the former surgeon's sex and cocaine addictions. Dr Wilcox said that he had, 'more time to think about how his addiction led to the destruction of his life and other lives as well. I believe now that he has been in custody for six months that denial has well and truly confronted. He has come to terms with the seriousness of his addiction and the consequences of his actions'.

On his own behalf, Nair said, 'I'm really saddened that these two very young girls that died could be caught up in my behaviour'.

But it was to no avail, as he was again denied bail due to the strength of his addiction and the likelihood that he would reoffend.

In the meantime, the HCCC undertook to review all surgery that had been performed at Nepean Public Hospital under the direction of Dr Nair, but at the time of writing, that report has yet to surface.

At the committal hearing, which took place at Sydney's Downing Centre Local Court, beginning on 6 December 2010, a number of other witnesses came forward and gave evidence in relation to this matter, including myself. I was amongst the last to give evidence, and was there to interpret the levels of drugs detected in the victims' blood samples.

A number of women connected to the sex industry, who had been clients of Mr Nair, gave evidence that on arrival at his residence he would greet them with a plate on which there were lines of cocaine and urge them to get 'coked up'. The court also heard that he encouraged the girls to insert rocks of cocaine in their anuses and vaginas, something that Victoria McIntyre did, although others refused.

A lot of the witnesses were concerned about the effects their appearing would have on their regular occupations and personal relationships, as they led double lives, so the crown prosecutor, Ms Kate Thompson, applied to have their names suppressed, saying it would cause damage to their careers and personal relationships if they were outed as former and current sex workers.

The police officers involved in the case, Detective Senior Constables Ben Tearne, Gavin Bradbury and Brad Semken provided testimony to corroborate the fears, but Magistrate Carolyn Barkell rejected all the applications except for one woman, Emily, who had since returned to the United States. She was subsequently cross-examined via audio-visual link and told the court that she'd been at Dr Nair's apartment at the time Victoria McIntyre had overdosed. She also said that she'd told Anna Monaghan, the director of HM International escort agency, that the group had been taking a lot of drugs and putting them into their orifices.

A medical expert from the Royal Prince Alfred Hospital emergency department, Dr Timothy Green, was called to give evidence. He told the court that Dr Nair would have recognised the warning signs of cocaine toxicity and should have called an ambulance when Suellen Domingues-Zaupa started suffering seizures. He further stated that a medic could have successfully treated her seizures, by intravenous medication.

Pathologists Rianie van Vuuren and Isabella Brouwer, who carried out the post-mortems on Victoria McIntyre and Suellen Domingues-Zaupa, also provided evidence regarding the same matter.

Dr Rianie van Vuuren was of the opinion that through the toxicology analysis and in the absence of any other symptoms in her body, she had died from cocaine toxicity.

I was the second last witness to give evidence and I was cross examined by Suresh Nair's barrister, Mr Peter Hamill, Senior Counsel, on a number of issues relating to cocaine ingestion, including levels of the drug found in the victims' blood samples, time of absorption, onset of effects and tolerance.

While the cocaine level in Suellen Domingues-Zaupa's blood had been very high at 4.9 milligrams per litre of blood and sufficient to cause death, Victoria McIntyre's cocaine concentration in her blood of 7.1 milligrams per litre had been truly extraordinary. I told the court it was probably one of the highest levels of cocaine I'd seen in my career.

Given that I had worked as a forensic scientist for more than thirty-two years, the last ten being with the NSW police (at the time of writing), it was no overstatement. Also, the administration of cocaine via the anus and vagina increases absorption of the drug and allows it to enter the bloodstream at a much greater rate, which would have accounted for the extreme cocaine levels detected in the victim's blood.

However, Mr Hamill pursued the issue of Victoria McIntyre's medical history and whether I had considered that when making my findings.

He then asked, 'Do you agree with the proposition that it is impossible and highly dangerous to speculate on the cause of death from cocaine based on toxicology alone?'

I replied, 'I generally prefer to base my findings on symptoms', and thought the elevated level of cocaine in Victoria McIntyre's blood had been more than sufficient to cause death, aside from any prior symptoms that may have been observed. [Cocaine concentrations in some thirty-seven recorded fatalities ranged from 0.04- 31 mg/L (average 4.6 mg/L). Both victims were well over this average level.]

The final committal hearing witness was Tanya Verhoeven, who was employed by Sydney Select Escorts at the time of Victoria McIntyre's death. She told the court Dr Nair had been a popular client with Sydney's escorts and that he liked girls who looked like models, lovely looking with good figures, but not too many curves. She also said that she would never have believed that as a doctor he would behave in such a dangerous manner. Further questioning revealed that Tanya had organised for Juliette Lancaster to attend Dr Nair's Valentine's Day party at his apartment on the fateful 15 February, and that Juliette had phoned her later that evening to tell her that there were police cars everywhere and that something had happened.

Suresh Nair subsequently appeared before Judge Robert Toner at Sydney District Court for sentencing on 26 August 2011. He'd initially been accused of two offences: the murder of Suellen Domingues-Zaupa in November 2009 and the manslaughter of fellow escort Victoria McIntyre in February, 2009, both women having been supplied with cocaine at his Elizabeth Bay apartment.

In a plea bargain carve-up, both charges were reduced markedly. Suresh Nair pleaded guilty to the manslaughter of Suellen Domingues-Zaupa and the murder charge was dropped, and guilty to supplying cocaine to Victoria McIntyre and her manslaughter charge was dropped.

Prior to sentencing, Judge Toner heard complimentary references from former patients of Dr Nair and a glowing testimony from leading brain surgeon, Dr Charlie Teo.

Judge Toner commented, 'It's hard to underestimate the fall of the prisoner. I find this evidence powerful and, at the same time, difficult to reconcile with the man who committed these crimes, where he essentially abandoned his sense of responsibility. Such, though, are the contradictions in this profoundly sad case'.

He then sentenced Nair to a maximum of nine years gaol, with a non-parole period of five years and four months. As he had been in custody since January 2010, he was eligible for parole on 30 April 2015.

However, he never did serve his full sentence.

In 2013, his prison term was reduced on appeal, and in July 2014, he became eligible for parole after serving less than three years in gaol. That was extraordinary given his history and the lead up to the death of Victoria McIntyre, when a disturbing warning had been circulated among all commercial sex establishments identifying him as a violent client who had almost killed a sex worker. Only a few short weeks later, Victoria McIntyre met her death at the hands of Nair, followed by Suellen Domingues-Zaupa, who died in his apartment after a similar incident. The gaol sentence he received was clearly inadequate given the offences.

But the case of Suresh Surendranath Nair didn't end there.

Mr Scott Morrison had recently been appointed as Immigration Minister, and he took his duties very seriously.

Although Suresh Nair had lived in Australia since he'd been a child, he'd never taken up citizenship, and because of his crimes, he was deregistered.

Mr Morrison cancelled his resident visa on 30 July 2014, on the grounds of character, so when Nair was released from Silverwater prison on 31 July, he was taken to the detention centre at Villawood and subsequently deported to back to Malaysia, where he'd been born.

So the classmate who wrote in the yearbook, next to Nair's photograph, wasn't far wrong in his prediction when he said that by 2011 he would be deregistered and exiled to the rainforests of the Amazon to live with cannibals. At least, he escaped the rainforests of the Amazon to live with cannibals, although in an extraordinary turn of events, it transpired that in the lead-up to his conviction, Nair had applied for Australian citizenship, but the paperwork had never been processed.

Could the tragic events that unfolded have been prevented? Possibly.

Very few people get *three* chances to sort out their lives before it impacts upon their career choice and other lives in the community. Unfortunately, Dr Nair had the luck of the devil in that he slipped through cracks in the system and was still able to practise medicine in spite of his first two suspensions and abundant evidence of his drug usage. Several of his colleagues expressed concern about him returning to work after yet another suspension, yet in his seemingly charmed life, he was allowed to return to work for a third time, albeit under supervision.

So, who was responsible for the impaired doctor? The Medical Board? The doctor's supervisor and/or employer? Or the Health Care Complaints Commission?

In reality, probably all of them. With better communication, the true nature of the doctor's problems would have been known and appropriate preventative action could have been taken.

Were lessons learned from this case?

Hopefully, yes, for all professionals concerned and for the better treatment any future patients that may come under the 'care' of an impaired doctor.

14

Death of a Dancer: A Deadly Drug Mistake

'Dancing faces you towards Heaven, whichever direction you turn.'

~Terri Guillemets

The subjective effects of MDMA (or 3, 4 - methylenedioxymethylamphetamine) have contributed to its popularity as a party drug among adolescents and young adults who attend rave or rock parties. It's known by a variety of names, the most recognised one amongst the general public being ecstasy, as that is how it's referred to in the news media whenever it features in a story. However, you may also have heard of XTC, Vitamin E and ADAM.

Whatever it's called, it's used recreationally for its stimulant and hallucinogenic effects, which combine the effects of mescaline and amphetamine. The drug has no approved medical use in Australia, but is widely abused. The most common methods of taking MDMA are orally (generally in tablet form), nasally (by snorting), by intra-venous injection and via suppositories. MDMA is rapidly absorbed when taken orally (the usual method of ingestion), but injecting has been reported as having the quickest onset and producing a more intense but shorter lasting experience. The effect of taking larger doses has been reported as mainly hallucinatory, with increasingly undesirable side effects occurring as the dose is ramped up. The onset of action of the drug is usually within thirty to forty minutes and a maximal response is achieved in about one or two hours. The duration of action is about four to six hours (mean five hours) and the drug and its metabolites are excreted mainly in the urine.

The negative effects of ecstasy are dose-related, in that their severity correlates with both the total number of doses consumed and the frequency of use. Short-term high dose use of MDMA has produced incidences of an amphetamine-like psychosis and, in some cases, severe hyperthermia that becomes unresponsive to medical intervention, leading to death.

Those properties are bad enough, but now a more deadly dark cousin drug of MDMA is lurking in the wings. Known as para-methoxy-amphetamine or PMA, it's one of a group of methoxylated phenethylamine derivatives or so-called designer drugs with marked hallucinogenic properties. PMA has about five times the potency of the naturally occurring drug mescaline. Hyperpyrexia (elevated body temperature), agitation (fidgeting), tachycardia (racing heartbeat), shallow laboured breathing and hypertension (elevated blood pressure) are common symptoms of over dosage.

PMA is a highly toxic amphetamine drug, which is often passed off as ecstasy, and it's been linked to a number of deaths in Australia and overseas. It's managed to infiltrate the drug scene mostly because it has been easier to obtain than the precursor chemicals for the synthesis of 3, 4-methylenedioxymethylamphetamine. The psychoactive effects of PMA have a slower onset than MDMA, which PMA is often sold as, and that being the case, the increased effects and slower onset can create a very dangerous situation for users by encouraging consumption of larger quantities of the drug.

With her infectious smile and cheeky nature, Annabel Catt could get away with almost anything. Her brother, Anthony, recalled that she could persuade almost anyone with a special combination of straight honesty and a cheeky smile on her face.

Her true passion was dancing. At the age of twenty, she was a part-time dance teacher at an Avalon dance school and had been at the Brent Street performing arts school for six years. Dancing was an important part of her life. Her mother, Alison, said that even when she played basketball or netball, she danced across the court.

On 17 February 2007, she went to the Good Vibrations Festival, or GVF, as it's often called. The GVF began in 2003 and has now become a landmark event in the Australian summer calendar. The day was warm and sunny and everyone appeared to be in good spirits, keen to listen and dance to some top musical acts. That year, some of the headline makers were the Beastie Boys, Snoop Dogg, Timo Maas, Nightmares on Wax, Jurassic 5, Cassius, Rhazel, DJ JS-One, Thunderball, DJ Yoda, Fort Knox Five, DJ Dan, Cut Copy, Cicada, Ursula 1000 and Kraak & Smaak.

The festival in Sydney's Centennial Park drew a crowd of thirty-two thousand, which caused the drug dealers present to rub their hands in glee. It was a veritable candy shop for revellers looking to buy.

Annabel was in her element, mixing with friends and generally having a good time. She loved the variety of music almost as much as the dancing. At about 2 pm, as the music blared out, she took a break and sat down on the grass with a group of her friends to pop a tablet of ecstasy. The drugs had been supplied by the boyfriend of her friend, Bodene Sheed, who'd put six ecstasy tablets and six capsules of MDMA in a plastic bag; the latter drug supposedly being a powder form of ecstasy. The bag containing the drugs was duly passed around and everyone helped themselves.

After a couple of hours, Annabel and one of her friends, Danielle Lettoof, took another ecstasy tablet, and then, with the effects of the first tablet wearing off, both decided to take an MDMA capsule. Sometime later, leaving the festival and feeling no reaction, Annabel took a second capsule. As she and her friends were travelling home on the bus, they began to hallucinate and sweat and find it difficult to walk properly. Annabel started to experience further adverse effects of the drugs and her leg muscles went into spasms, knocking the seat in front of her. Her arms tightened and veins popped out. On reaching Mona Vale, she was helped into her home, suffering from hyperthermia. As her temperature was so high, her friends thought a shower should do the trick and cool her down, which it did temporarily.

By that stage, she was becoming a bit agitated, but so were the other girls, so they decided the best course of action was to go to bed and sleep it off. During the night Annabel began to suffer much worse. The spasms in her legs caused her to kick a chest of drawers at the foot of her bed, and the noise woke her companions, who turned on the light and realised that not only was she having difficulty breathing, but she had also turned an 'eerie ice blue'.

Her friend, Danielle Lettoof, was exhibiting similar symptoms, but was not as severely affected. However, her eyes were extremely dilated and she was also showing physical signs of hyperthermia. An ambulance was called and the two young women were rushed off to hospital, arriving at the intensive care unit in just eight minutes, at 5.30 am. Annabel's body temperature was 41.9 degrees Celsius; a dangerously high temperature given the body's normal temperature is 37.5 degrees Celsius. An ice bag was applied to lower her temperature and she was intubated.

Danielle had not taken a second MDMA capsule, as she had become physically ill about an hour after taking the first one, and had warned the others not to take theirs because of her reaction. However, the drug was still affecting her, as she was pale, her eyes were extremely dilated and she was showing physical signs of hyperthermia. Even so, she was still lucid and able to inform police that she and Annabel had taken an MDMA cap each, which had been purchased from Bodene Sheed.

In the meantime, the medical staff were making heroic efforts to save Annabel's life. They administered midazolam to reduce the seizures and spasms, gave her electric shocks to get her heart back into rhythm and ventilated her to aid her breathing. But, it was a losing battle. Had she gone to hospital sooner, the outcome may have been quite different, but at 6.13 am, Annabel passed away. Her friend, Danielle, survived.

A blood sample taken from Annabel at the autopsy was found to contain MDMA 0.5 milligrams per litre, midazolam less than 0.1 milligrams per litre and 4-methoxyamphetamine (or para-methoxyamphetamine, or PMA) 1.9 milligrams per litre. I found the level of MDMA in her blood to be particularly high given the therapeutic range is 0.1 – 0.35 milligrams per litre for the feel good, euphoric effects sought by users of the drug, and that indicated several tablets had been taken. But more important was the level of PMA, which was well within the lethal range. That indicated a very high dosage (there is no theraputic level range for this drug, however, a number of fatalities resulting from oral or intravenous (injected) use of PMA had postmortem blood levels ranging from 0.3 to 1.9 milligrams per litre and even higher). The remaining capsule was given to the police, who had it analysed and found it contained a very high content of PMA, at 44.5 per cent. As I indicated in my subsequent statement: 'The level of PMA in Ms Catt's blood would have been more than sufficient to result in her death, even without the additive effects from MDMA.'

Annabel's death struck a deep chord within the community. Grief counselling was provided to the friends who were with her on the fateful day, and all were encouraged to seek ongoing trauma/grief counselling.

On 21 February 2007, Bodene Sheed of Mona Vale was charged at Dee Why police station with supplying a prohibited drug, namely PMA and ecstasy, at the Good Vibrations Festival. She was granted conditional bail to appear at the Manly Local Court on 21 March 2007. The matter was subsequently moved to the Downing Centre Local Court, where Bodene Sheed appeared before Magistrate Robert Williams for sentencing. Members of the Catt family were not present.

Bodene Sheed pleaded guilty to two counts of supplying a prohibited drug, namely six tablets of ecstasy and six MDMA capsules.

In his opening address, his Honour said it was clear the offence had had a tragic result that Ms Sheed may not have been able to foresee, but that the difficulty in the matter was that that was what had happened. It could not have been a more tragic result, but he was sure that that had been brought home to her.

Bodene Sheed's barrister, Mr Anthony Jamieson, described his client as deeply remorseful, and said she'd made no money from the supply, merely passing on the bag of tablets which had been obtained from another person. In addition, he said, 'All of the girls had freely been using drugs'.

His Honour Williams noted Ms Sheed's remorse, the fact that those she had supplied had used drugs before and that the drug supply had not been a large one. However, he noted, it had played a significant part in the tragedy and it was important that a message be sent to the community that Parliament and the courts were against the supply of drugs in any quantity. He continued to say that it was beholden on him to recognise the harm done to the victim and to the community.

Detective Sergeant Stephen Pollard, who investigated the case, told the magistrate that there had been no other arrests in relation to the matter and that the defendant had been very forthcoming, supplying information that was to the best of her knowledge.

Magistrate Robert Williams said although Bodene Sheed couldn't have known the tragic consequences that would unfold, she still had to take responsibility for her actions. He then sentenced her to a hundred and twenty hours of community service.

Bodene Sheed shed tears in the box, and nodded as Magistrate Williams warned another slip up would leave her in jail.

Outside the court, Ms Sheed was asked by reporters if she was remorseful over her friend's death, and whether she would never use drugs again. She replied in the affirmative to both questions before being driven away.

Mrs Alison Catt somewhat generously told ABC radio that she believed Ms Bodene Sheed was also a victim.

'We see her as another victim really', she said. 'She was the foot soldier in this and we're glad she has been able to help the police with further investigations. I think why it's been reported so widely is because we are an ordinary family and she was just a fun loving, ordinary girl and she wasn't into drugs, so this can happen to anyone.'

Mrs Catt concluded that she hoped lessons would be learnt from her daughter's death.

Annabel father, Peter, said, 'We really wish that if anything positive comes out of the loss of our dear Annabel, it is that other people would think twice before taking any kind of drug'.

The question as to why Annabel Catt died while her companion, Danielle Lettoof survived was asked, and the answer lies in the dosages of the drugs taken. Danielle only took one capsule, while Annabel took two. That probably contributed to Danielle's reaction to the drug, which while serious, was not fatal. Had she consumed that other capsule containing the PMA, the final outcome would most likely have been even more tragic, with the deaths of two young people.

15
The Antique Knife

'Alcohol appears a friend, it lulls you in,
but too much of it, can make you sin.'
~ Anon

Chiam Kimel met Danielle Stewart at a Kings Cross nightclub. He was forty-nine and she was twenty-four, but love was blind to the age difference and they got married three years later. A year after, they started an online catering company, The Epicurian, with a thirty thousand dollar loan from Danielle's doting grandmother, Elaine Craker. They lived in rented accommodation on New South Head Road, Rose Bay. It was on the fourth floor of the complex and had two bedrooms, the second one being occupied by Jordan Kimel, Chiam's son from a previous relationship, who was ten years old when Chiam and Danielle first met. Chiam's two other children, Amber and Fred, were older and lived their own independent lives.

However, life wasn't a bed of roses, as Danielle suffered from a history of mental illness and self-harm, which led to various domestic issues and screaming matches, but for the next three years they soldiered on, living through a marriage that could be tumultuous and unpredicatable because of Danielle's mood swings.

On the evening of 23 August 2006, Danielle and Chiam went out to dinner with their friends, Angela Batley and Harley Nash, at the Pescador Fish and Grill Restaurant in New South Head Road, Rose Bay. They arrived at 7 pm, were seated immediately and ordered their drinks and dinner.

During the course of the meal, they consumed two bottles of wine. It was a pleasant setting, and good-natured banter flowed amongst the party. At 8.30 pm, the waitress fetched the bill and placed it on their table.

Angela commented, 'The best thing about this restaurant is the chips', to which Danielle replied, moving her hand towards the waitress, 'The best thing about this restaurant is you'. The alcohol had begun to talk, although Angela said later in a gross understatement, 'Nobody seemed too badly affected by alcohol, although we were fairly jolly'.

True, they were all in a good mood, and the plan was to drive to Angela and Harley's place to have a few more drinks and further conversation. However, Danielle drove her car back to her and Chiam's apartment, while Chiam went back to their friend's place. At the time Angela, Harley and Chiam thought she was taking her dog, 'Echo', home, which was in the car. However, when she showed up at Angela and Harley's unit a little later, she still had the dog with her.

While they sat around chatting, Danielle consumed more red wine, and as the evening wore on, she started getting a bit moody and argumentative with Chiam. They stayed for a couple of hours, and when Chiam remarked, 'It's lovely to be surrounded by happy, healthy people', Danielle replied, 'What if we aren't healthy? It isn't practical in everyday life'.

The couple then left in Danielle's car, arriving home at about 11 pm. Danielle said to Chiam's son, 'I shouldn't have gone. I've had too much to drink'. She then walked into the kitchen, put down her handbag and took out her iPod before retreating to the living area of the apartment to play some music through the computer speakers. A little while later, Chiam came into the room with Jordan and asked her to turn down the volume because it would be disturbing the neighbours. She did, but then immediately turned it back up again. A disgusted Jordan left the scene and went to his bedroom, shutting the door. Chiam then turned the volume down again and Danielle responded by turning it back up. That occurred a number of times and developed into an argument which became louder and more aggressive.

Danielle shouted, 'You fucking barred me out of the computer. You fucking barred me out of the computer'. Then she punched him

'There's no need to get violent', Chiam replied, trying to take the sting out of the situation.

But Danielle was not to be pacified. She reached for the antique knife which they kept on the coffee table and unsheathed it.

'What are you doing?' Chiam exclaimed. 'Are you crazy?'

He then screamed in pain three times as Danielle plunged it into his body. Jordan came running in to be confronted by an awful sight. His father had his left hand against the wall, holding himself up, and his right hand across his left rib cage. His white shirt was covered in blood. He looked at his son and said, 'She stabbed me. She stabbed me. Call the ambulance'.

Danielle was standing opposite Chiam, holding the antique knife in her right hand. There was blood on her fingers. The sheaf that the knife was normally kept in was in her left hand. She was crying. 'You fucking barred me out of the internet,' she said.

When Jordan went back into his room to fetch his mobile phone, she followed him, screaming, 'Get the fuck out. Get the fuck out,' all the while motioning towards the door with the knife in her hand.

'You fucking stabbed my father!' Jordan shouted.

But precious moments were ebbing away, as indeed was Chiam's life. Jordan quickly put on some shorts and thongs and ran out into the hallway outside the apartment, where he knocked on the front door of a neighbour. Josh Mathew opened it.

‘Please help,’ Jordan pleaded. ‘My father’s been stabbed.’

Josh, his brother Daniel and Jordan charged down the hall to help Chiam, who was now lying in front of the elevator with a mobile phone to his ear. There was blood everywhere.

Jordan headed back down the hallway to get some more help from other neighbours. As he did, Danielle stormed out of the apartment holding the knife, the sheaf and a computer flat screen monitor.

‘I stabbed him! I stabbed him!’ she shouted. ‘Look what he’s done to me!’

She then dropped the computer monitor on the floor and threw the blood stained antique knife and its sheaf down the stairs before going back into the apartment.

In the meantime, Jordan returned to his father, who was still on the mobile phone to an operator. Josh, Daniel and Jordan laid him down in the elevator and took him down to the ground floor.

‘Call the ambulance. Call the ambulance,’ Chiam kept saying.

Jordan took the mobile off his father and spoke to the operator, giving her the address, which was also relayed to the police. The operator advised Jordan to get a clean cloth and put pressure on his father’s wounds. Chiam was now in a very bad way and struggling for life.

Jordan placed a cushion under his head and tried to calm him by saying, ‘Don’t talk. Breathe deeply. Try not to move’.

‘I love you very much’, Chiam whispered. ‘Everything is going to be alright.’

The situation was quickly becoming more than Jordan could handle. He felt a surge of uncontrollable anger and ran into the laundry, grabbing a golf club. When he came back out, he brandished it over his head, declaring, ‘I’m gonna kill her!’

Fortunately, he was restrained by Josh and Daniel, who calmed him down and told him to be strong. Jordan then went outside to gather himself together.

While he was there, the police arrived, so he went back inside the building and sat by his father, waiting for the ambulance.

'Danielle…' Chiam gasped, clutching a blood soaked towel to his abdomen.

The ambulance arrived and Chiam was loaded onto a stretcher and taken to St Vincent's Hospital for emergency surgery, where he died on the operating table later that night. It was now a case of murder.

With Chiam on his way to hospital, the police went upstairs to find Danielle

It wasn't difficult, as a thick trail of blood covering the carpet of the communal floor and splattering the walls led them to the couple's front door. They also saw the antique knife with blood on its handle at the bottom of the stairs in the common area of the building, with its sheaf lying nearby. Outside the apartment, they observed the computer flat screen monitor, splattered in blood, along with numerous receipts and various pieces of paperwork.

After getting no response to requests to open up, they forced entry, but on gaining access to the apartment, a curious sight befell them. Danielle was sitting on a couch, holding an iPod, notepad and pen.

'Are you Danielle?' Sergeant Richard Lord asked.

'Are you Danielle?' she mimicked in response.

Sergeant Lord then took the iPod, pen and pad from Danielle and asked, 'Where's the knife?'

'What knife?' she replied, before adding, 'But I was studying!'

Sergeant Lord then explained her rights, to which she quipped, 'My rights? Really? That's funny because you're in my house'.

While Sergeant Lord was talking to Danielle, another police officer searched the apartment, discovering a blister pack of Seroquel (a brand of quetiapine) tablets under her bed. Nineteen tablets were missing.

Danielle was arrested and handcuffed, but she refused to walk, so three police officers had to carry her to the police cage truck. She kicked and screamed all the way down to the wagon, yelling out to her sixteen-year-old stepson, who was not present, 'How could you do this to me? After all I did for you! How could you betray me like this?'

Once in the back of the wagon, she lay motionless on the floor and bumps were heard each time the wagon turned the corner. She was clearly incapacitated and so it was fairly bumpy journey. However, due to her bizarre behaviour, which alternated between lucid to irrational, she was later transferred to an ambulance, which took her to the Prince of Wales Hospital to obtain blood samples. She was accompanied by Constable Julie-Anne Johnson.

On arrival at the hospital, Danielle turned to her and yelled. 'Bitch! Bitch!'

She also abused the doctors and nurses trying to calm her. 'Don't you fucking touch me, you bitch.' Then she fumed, 'He wouldn't let me into the computer. He's taken all the money I put into my business. He's ruined my business. I want to call my grandmother. I have no mother or father. Please let me call her. I don't have anyone. He's probably sitting at home fucking laughing at me'.

Eventually, blood samples were obtained and forwarded for analysis to the Division of Analytical Laboratories at Lidcombe.

Danielle was assessed both physically and psychologically before being discharged at 4 pm, when she was taken to Waverly police station, where she was entered into custody and read her rights. She was subsequently charged, and due to the circumstances, taken into custody.

On 7 July 2008, she stood trial at the NSW Supreme Court in Taylor Square, Darlinghurst for the murder Chiam Kimel on the evening of the 23 August 2006.

A number of issues were raised during the trial, including Danielle's personality disorder, which supposedly caused her to live in constant fear that Mr Kimel would leave her.

Poignantly, Danielle's grandmother, Ms Elaine Kraker, was asked if the two loved each other, to which she replied, 'Yes, and that's what I can't understand'.

It was also revealed that less than a month after murdering her husband,

Danielle had written to his best friend and former lover, Angela Batley, saying:

For really the first time in our relationship, everything was really good between Chiam and I. Apart from a few hiccups we were closer to each other than we had ever been.

On page three of the letter she wrote:

> I'm so sorry, it should be me that's dead. I never meant to hurt Chiam, let alone kill him. There is not one single part of me that wants him dead. I want him alive. I want my life back. I want our life back. He was my best friend. I have nothing without him. I woke one day with a beautiful life, then woke up three days later in hell. I am so traumatised knowing what this has done to his children. I love Jordan as if he was my own flesh and blood. I'm so worried that he doesn't have Chiam now, that he may have to live with Diana who doesn't give a shit about him really. Chiam was my whole life, as I know I was his whole life.

During the trial, further revelations about their stormy relationship were revealed.

Dr Rosalind Foy, who had treated Danielle for about five months before she fatally stabbed her husband with the antique knife, told the Supreme Court jury that Danielle suffered from a borderline personality disorder, similar to a post-traumatic stress disorder, as a result of being sexually abused by a number of people as a child. She went on to describe her as being deeply disturbed in an angry fashion with a high level of anxiety.

It wasn't just her childhood trauma that was raised, but also an abortion that had left her feeling depressed and suicidal. Dr Foy said it had been very distressing for her. However, the pregnancy hadn't been due to her husband.

Danielle had become pregnant by another lover, whose name was given as Yuri Moel, when she'd visited in Melbourne during a brief separation from Chiam during 2005.

Dr Foy told the court that Yuri had wanted to keep the child and have her live with him in Melbourne, while Chiam had told her to have a termination if she wanted to stay with him. In the event, Danielle had decided it was not the time to be having children.

Danielle's barrister, Belinda Rigg, suggested that Chiam was '… dominating and controlling and she'd get defensive and angry and they'd fight', and Danielle claimed that on the night of the stabbing, she was acting in self-defence and that her husband had been physically violent towards her.

However, that was at odds with the evidence presented by Dr Foy, who denied Danielle had mentioned physical abuse at the hands of Chiam during their lengthy sessions, although she had said she had difficulties with his personality. 'She would say she wasn't happy with him. She was feeling isolated. They didn't socialise very much and they didn't have common friends except Angela (Bately), who was always miserable and who was an ex-partner of her husband.'

Further evidence was presented by Chiam's daughter, Mrs Amber Rubenstein, who told the court that her father was a gentle giant who had been abused by Danielle. She said that Danielle had bitten him on the thumb and arm a number of times, and had smashed or damaged his glasses so often that it had become a running joke in the family that he had to get his glasses replaced regularly.

A damaged set of glasses had been found in the apartment on the night of the stabbing, which seemed to back up that claim.

Mrs Rubenstein went on to tell the court that she'd seen Danielle in happy moods and that she was lovely. She also said that she'd really liked her until she'd seen her aggressive outbursts for herself.

In a further revelation, she said that when she and her brother, Fred Kimel, had been cleaning out the home that Chiam had shared with Danielle, they had come across a draft of a play written by Danielle about a woman who plots her husband's violent murder.

'I couldn't believe my eyes', Mrs Rubenstein said, with tears in her eyes. 'I was horrified and tormented by these revelations. After reading her writings I felt cheated – I didn't know she had thoughts like this. There is a synopsis of a play in which one of the characters has secret desires to kill her husband in a violent rage. There are study notes on jail architecture, prisoner psychology, different cell classifications, prison attire, prison visiting hours and life sentences.'

Fred Kimel commented, 'How am I able to understand how someone could have perpetrated such a crime having already considered the potential ramifications?'

However, the unfinished manuscript was not allowed as evidence in the trial because there was uncertainty as to Danielle's sobriety (due to drugs and/or alcohol) at the time of writing.

A number of other witnesses came forward and gave evidence in relation to this latter matter, including me. I was there to interpret the levels of drugs and alcohol found in Danielle's blood, and so determine to what level she would have been affected at the time of the incident. The analyst's reports (carried out by the Division of Analytical Laboratories, Lidcombe, New South Wales and the Victorian Institute of Forensic Medicine, Southbank, Victoria) showed that she had the following levels of drugs and alcohol in her blood:

- diazepam 0.06 – 0.08 milligrams per litre,
- nordiazepam <0.01 milligrams per litre,
- temazepam <0.01 milligrams per litre,
- quetiapine 1.3 milligrams per litre, and
- alcohol 0.203 grams per decilitre (100 millilitres) of blood.

Of those, the most important were the levels of the quetiapine and alcohol. Quetiapine is available under the trade name of Seroquel, an Astra Zeneca product, and is an antipsychotic drug which has been shown to be effective in the treatment of schizophrenia. Danielle had indicated earlier that on the evening of the incident, she'd taken nearly a whole packet of Seroquel, crushing some of the tablets into soya milk before drinking them. While the level of quetiapine detected was significant (just over double the top end of therapeutic range), the major player was alcohol.

I estimated the level of alcohol in her blood at the time of the incident to most likely be at 0.240 per cent and concluded that,' given the estimated blood alcohol level and the elevated level of quetiapine present in her blood at the time of the incident, her ability to think rationally about her actions would have been compromised'. A similar estimation of her blood alcohol at the time of the incident was confirmed by other experts. Dr Graham Starmer further described the alcohol level at the time of the incident as swamping the effects of the other drugs.

By a majority verdict, the jury found that Danielle was not guilty of murdering her husband, but guilty of his manslaughter. Although Danielle said she'd been acting in self-defence when she'd stabbed Chiam in the stomach with the antique knife, the prosecution contended that there was no element of self-defence in her actions, arguing that she'd stabbed her husband in an argument over their catering business.

Sentencing took place on 16 December 2008. Acting Justice Jane Mathews made reference to Danielle's blood alcohol reading at the time of the stabbing, which had been calculated to be 0.240. She concluded that the combination of a high level of alcohol intoxication and Danielle's borderline personality disorder had led to the tragedy, and turning to Chiam's three children seated in the public gallery, said, 'I suspect that you'll regard the punishment that that I am about to impose as quite inadequate to the extent of your loss'.

However, she did add that no punishment would ever be able to redress their loss and that there were a number of factors to consider before delivering the sentence.

She then handed Danielle a maximum of six years and four months, with a minimum of four years gaol, backdating the conviction to when she was taken into custody.

By the time Danielle Stewart is released, she will have received appropriate treatment for her borderline personality disorder and, hopefully, also given up the alcohol. Otherwise, Fred Kimel's comment, 'I worry that if she is not able to take full responsibility for her actions (that) she will always present a threat', may well become a prophecy.

16

'Takeaway Morphine': The Dr Gow Case

'Poisons and medicine are often times the same substance given with different intents.'

~Peter Mere Latham

Morphine is the principal alkaloid of opium, the dried latex extracted by shallowly slicing the unripe seedpods of the *Papaver somniferum* poppy. It's used as a powerful opiate analgesic for the treatment of moderate to severe pain. As with other opioid analgesics, the main side effects are nausea, vomiting, drowsiness, constipation and respiratory depression. Tolerance to most of those usually develops with long-term usage, the exception being constipation due to reduced gastro-intestinal motility. As for dosage, the accepted level to treat pain in adults is five to twenty milligrams by injection, taken every four hours if needed. However, an individual with heightened reflex excitability of their nervous system may take two or three times the ordinary dose and suffer few, if any, side effects. For example, a patient with severe pain from renal colic or coronary disease may be given forty-five to sixty milligrams before pain relief is obtained, with no serious respiratory problems. Generally speaking, the toxic dose of morphine for a non-addicted person is somewhere in the region of sixty milligrams, and serious symptoms are usually experienced after doses of a hundred milligrams, resulting in increased respiratory depression and consequent anoxia (a total lack of oxygen).

Wayne Neil Ritchie, fifty-two years old and retired from the Australian Army, was afflicted with chronic back pain as a result of suffering a back injury a number of years earlier. His condition was further exacerbated as a result of a fall from a one-tonne truck while moving furniture, although he didn't seek any medical treatment after the accident.

He shared a two-storey brick premises on Brentwood Avenue, Figtree with a female friend, Andrea Sant. The premises became known as the Brahma Kumaris Raja Yoga Meditation Centre, where they regularly conducted meetings on yoga and meditation. The pair became close friends through the organisation, telling people they were like brother and sister and spiritual partners, and they became engaged to be married.

Richie learned to live with his chronic back pain by taking doses of Panadeine Forte and Codalgin Forte (both strong codeine and paracetamol formulations), which were prescribed by his physician, Dr Mackay. At the same time, Andrea was receiving pethidine for pain associated with her genetic medical condition so it's possible she may have shared her meds with him. Whether she did or not, we don't know, but what we do know is that Richie started to develop a tolerance to his and wanted something more effective. He tried to persuade his regular doctor to prescribe him a stronger painkiller, such as morphine, but he refused, so Andrea suggested that he try Dr Gary Gow, who had a homeopathic practice in Church Street, Wollongong. He initially suggested some herbal remedies, but when they proved to be unsuccessful, he agreed to Richie's request for morphine, writing out a prescription for morphine tartrate 120 mg/1.5 ml (x 5 pack) ampoules.

The prescription read:

ars 30

podo 30

morphine tartrate 5 120mg

The *ars* refers to arsenic albumen, while *podo* is podophyllum, both of which are homeopathic remedies for traveller's diarrhoea.

Dr Gow had intended to prescribe morphine sulphate, which was available at a maximum strength of 30 mg/1.0 ml, in a pack of five ampoules, but on hearing from Richie that he and Andrea were planning to travel to India and that he was worried about managing his back pain during the flight, he became momentarily confused and made a mistake, prescribing the wrong drug.

The prescription was presented at a Figtree pharmacy, which had no stock of morphine tartrate and had to order it in, duly dispensing it to Richie on 29 September 2004.

When Richie awoke on the morning of 2 October, he was suffering from both neck and back pain. At about 10 am, he had a two-hour massage, which gave him some relief, and then engaged in some meditation. But as the day progressed, the pain became unrelenting. As it intensified into the evening, it looked like stronger treatment was needed.

At 7 pm, Richie decided it was time to get some pain relief and the sleep that went with it, so he asked Andrea to help him with the morphine, as he had difficulty with the glass ampoules. She opened one of them and filled the syringe with the amount prescribed. Looking at the strength of the morphine (120mg/1.5mL), she commented that it was a lot stronger than the pethidine. She then handed the syringe to Richie, who injected himself in his right thigh.

Following the injection, the two of them chatted until Richie said he could already feel the drug working and that he wanted to go to sleep. By 7.30 pm, he was snoring, so Andrea also turned in, waking at 4 am to do her meditation, after which she returned to bed before waking again at around 6 am to make some breakfast. She checked on Richie a couple of times and everything appeared to be okay, but on the third time, she became aware that the room was silent. Richie had stopped snoring. On closer inspection, she saw that there wasn't only vomit on the mattress, but also sweat on Richie's head.

He was lying on his side and she was unable to roll him over onto his back, so she rang for an ambulance. While she was waiting, she had another, more successful, attempt at rolling him onto his back. Immediately, she began CPR and kept at it until the ambulance officers arrived a short time later, when they took over. Unfortunately, there was nothing they could do for Richie, and they told Andrea that he was dead. When they asked her about any medications he might have taken, she showed them the packet of morphine ampoules. The paramedics were most concerned, with one of them commenting, 'It would be enough to kill a horse!'

The police were informed and, a short time later, Wollongong detectives, general duties police and a crime scene officer arrived at the address. Upon examination of the body, it was observed that Richie's finger tips and nails had turned dark blue, indicating anoxia. There was no sign of rigor mortis, blood pooling (an indication of a recent death), or signs of bruising on his body. His body was conveyed by ambulance to Wollongong Hospital, where his life was pronounced extinct at 10.22 am on 3 October by Dr Lee.

A blood sample taken at the autopsy was found to contain morphine 1.0 mg/L, and a bile sample taken at the same time was found to have a morphine level of greater than 40 mg/L of blood. That indicated a large amount of morphine had been taken, and that some time had elapsed before death had occurred from severe central nervous system depression (CNS), at which point, life was no longer sustainable.

The usual dosage for chronic pain is initially twenty milligrams of morphine every twelve hours or forty milligrams every twenty-four hours. As stated in the introduction to this story, in general, the toxic dose of morphine for a non-addicted person who is not in pain is about sixty milligrams, and serious symptoms are generally experienced after doses of a hundred milligrams. The outlook becomes less favourable as the amount increases, with death occurring as a result of marked respiratory depression and consequent anoxia. The injection containing a hundred and twenty milligrams of morphine as the tartrate salt was more than enough to take Richie's life.

In my report, I concluded that I was of the opinion that the morphine dosage was excessive and the subsequent blood level achieved in a non-tolerant person was more than sufficient to produce marked respiratory depression and consequent anoxia, resulting in death. A compromised respiratory condition (early bronchopneumonia) would have further exacerbated the condition.

The latter symptom could have been brought about by the CNS depressant effect of the morphine - one effect worsening the effect of another.

The police visited Dr Gow's surgery at 10.10 am on 5 October, in relation to the prescription for morphine tartrate provided by him to Richie.

'Come in', Dr Gow said. 'I was expecting you.'

'We're here in relation to one of your patients, Wayne Richie.'

'Yes, I know', Dr Gow replied. 'I know what happened. I made a mistake. I feel responsible for his death. I prescribed too much. I should have explained to him how much to use.'

Dr Gow was very remorseful and was advised to seek some legal advice from the medical union.

'Yes, maybe I should', he said. 'I made a mistake. It was clear on the prescription what was prescribed.'

Police informed him that the matter would be investigated and advice would be sought from the coroner in relation to procedures to be adopted. After further conversation about Richie's medical records, they returned to Wollongong police station.

At that juncture, the prosecution would only have been able to establish that Richie had been prescribed a hundred and twenty milligrams of morphine and that he'd died as a result of injecting that amount. Evidence was needed to show that the amount prescribed was excessive. What appeared to be a simple mistake followed by a drug over dosage – with a fatal result - needed to be proven. It had to be shown that the amount prescribed was 'grossly excessive' for the prosecution to commence. I advised that that was indeed the case, and on viewing Richie's medical records and factoring in the other opiates he'd taken, in particular Codalgin Forte, a strong pain-relief preparation containing codeine, I concluded that his opiate tolerance was minimal.

It was deemed that there was sufficient evidence to proceed, and Dr Gow was committed to stand trial in Wollongong's Local Court for the manslaughter of Richie.

Detective Senior Constable Frank Sanvitale said that the ambulance officers who had attended the scene had expressed concerns about the dosage of morphine that had been prescribed.

'One of them colourfully told you it was a dose that could kill a horse, is that right?' defence barrister Ms Elizabeth Fullerton asked.

'Yes, that's correct', Sanvitale replied.

I also testified at the initial trial on 3 April, 2006, and said that the usual dosage of morphine would be twenty milligrams over a twelve hour period or forty milligrams over twenty-four hours. I mentioned that severe side effects could be expected for any single dosage above sixty milligrams and that the central nervous system would start to shut down at one hundred milligrams. 'This (one hundred and twenty milligrams) is a very large amount and the only thing I can perceive it to be used for is in a hospital where respiration assistance would be available.'

When further cross-examined by Ms Fullerton, I conceded that I'd only recently learnt that one hundred and twenty milligrams had been the smallest dosage of morphine tartrate available at the pharmacy.

Ms Fullerton then asked, 'Does it surprise you then that the drug in that concentration is available to be dispensed to a walking, talking person on presentation of a prescription to a residential pharmacy?'

I replied, 'It horrifies me. It's just like take-away methadone. I totally disagree with it. It should be consumed on (medical) premises and administered by a qualified (medical) practitioner'.

Prior to my evidence, Ms Andrea Sant had told the court that she had merely followed the directions on the packaging when filling the syringe for Richie. 'It said one hundred and twenty milligrams or as directed by your doctor.'

She acknowledged that she hadn't asked Richie about the doctor's instructions, but said she'd had no idea of the strength of the morphine, other than to say, 'It was a lot stronger than the pethidine'.

After two days of evidence, Magistrate Johnson found there was enough evidence to prove Dr Gow had breached his duty of care by prescribing a potent drug, morphine, and failing to instruct his patient on its use, and the case was to proceed before a jury in the district court. A date of May 15 was set, but was subsequently postponed to 7 August, and the venue was changed from Wollongong to the Downing Centre in Sydney.

The trial was presided over by Judge Berman. I also attended and was again cross- examined by Ms Fullerton and the Crown. Unsurprisingly, my answers were the same as those I'd given at the local court. However, Dr Gow surprised everyone by changing his initial plea, pleading guilty to manslaughter on the following Monday morning.

An earlier plea of guilty would have saved a number of witnesses, as well as the accused, a lot of inconvenience due to the move from Wollongong to Sydney. But he must have thought it was worth a chance.

In his summation, Judge Berman said he'd never come across such a case and that it was unique in Australian law. He then asked for assistance from both the Crown and defence with regard to sentencing, precisely because there had never been a precedent to which he could refer. He then set a date of 20 October for the delivery of his judgment.

Dr Gow subsequently received an eighteen month suspended sentence. However, the NSW Medical Board restricted him from prescribing Schedule 8 drugs of addiction, which includes morphine, and decreed that he was not to possess, supply or administer those drugs. They also found that the prescribing pharmacist had questions to answer, and they summoned both parties to appear before them to account for their actions and the fatal outcome.

However, other events were to occur before that happened.

In April 2007, Dr Gow was diagnosed with multiple myeloma, a progressive disease of the blood and bone marrow. This cancer has a poor prognosis, and he passed away on 2 April 2009.

It's likely that the stress of the five years since Wayne Richie's death, and in particular, the final three years when he'd been subject to the scrutiny of the courts, the NSW Medical Board and the media, helped to hasten his end.

Despite the controversy, the Illawarra Division of GPs CEO, Dr Andrew Dalley, said that Dr Gow would be fondly remembered. 'Gary will be remembered for his quiet demeanour and his sincere compassion towards his patients. His staff were devoted to him. (During the controversy) he received an enormous amount of support from his patients and from his staff.'

He was survived by his wife, Lucia (Apolloni) and two daughters, Alexandra and Olivia, and a service was held for him at the Nan Tien Temple, Berkeley, Wollongong, at 10.30 am the following Tuesday.

Sadly, this was a case where a number of checkpoints weren't observed or considered. The prescribing doctor in the case, Dr Gow, apparently didn't check his physician's desk reference to determine a suitable dosage of the medication for his patient, and the pharmacist didn't check the prescription with the doctor before filling it 'as directed by your doctor' to determine what directions were to be given to the patient. And last, but certainly not least, Wayne Richie's life could have been saved by early medical intervention, possibly as late as 6 am, with a shot of Narcan (naloxone), as he'd developed some tolerance to opiates (possibly from ingesting earlier codeine preparations) to have lasted as long as twelve hours after injecting the large dose of morphine.

The only positive to come out of the whole episode is that Wayne Richie is at peace and no longer in pain.

17

Death on the High Seas: The Dianne Brimble Case

'Life isn't fair. It's just fairer than death, that's all.'
~ ***William Goldman***

The morning of 23 September 2002 was humid and cloudy, with the thermometer hovering at around eighteen degrees. At midday, give or take a few minutes, a new load of passengers arrived at Sydney's Darling Harbour Wharf 8 to board the cruise ship, the *Pacific Sky*, for a cruise around the Pacific. Among them was Dianne Brimble, who was very excited because, after saving for two years, the day had finally arrived for her holiday of a lifetime.

Dianne, a divorced suburban mother of three children, worked full-time as a furniture store saleswoman in Brisbane, Queensland. She was accompanied by her twelve-year-old daughter, Tahlia Michell, her older sister and regular traveller, Alma Wood, and her daughter, Kari-Anne, also twelve years old. All four of them were going to share a cabin. The first port of call for the tourists was to be Noumea, scheduled for Thursday, 26 September. They couldn't wait.

Unbeknown to them, a number of male passengers, later to be known as the 'eight persons of interest' also boarded the ship. They were Mark Wilhelm, Matthew Slade, Dragan Losic, Petar 'Pete' Pantic, Sakaleros 'Charlie' Kambouris, Letterio 'Leo' Silvestri, Luigi Vitale and Ryan Kuchel, and together they were to have a major impact on Dianne and her holiday. As fate would have it, the eight men were staying in two cabins (D182 and D178 - across from each other) on the same corridor as Dianne and her party (D188).

They were all from Adelaide, all had somewhat 'colourful' backgrounds and all displayed anti-social behaviour from the moment the ship left port. At the time, Dragan Losic, a forty-one-year-old father of three, had twenty-seven convictions and two gaol sentences under his belt, one of three and a half years for drug offences. His many convictions included one for carrying an offensive weapon when he was twenty, and breaking and entering. He'd also beaten a rape charge at the age of eighteen. In 2001, he'd been placed on a good behaviour bond after pleading guilty to being in possession of one thousand, eight hundred and forty cannabis plants. Sakaleros Kambouris had written a character reference for the trial, in which he described Losic as a 'devoted father and family man who was trustworthy, reputable and a man of honour'.

Luigi Vitale had convictions for producing drugs, assault and possessing an unlicensed firearm.

Mark Wilhelm had allegedly admitted to having and taking the drug fantasy, a street name for the chemical, gamma-hydroxybutyrate (GHB).

Letterio, or Leo (as he preferred to be called) Silvestri was no stranger to the courts either. For example, he'd been charged with amphetamine possession on 12 September 2001, and had been convicted on a number of counts of fraud. On 2 February 2000, he'd pleaded guilty to sixteen counts of falsely obtaining social security benefits and had subsequently been given a four-month suspended sentence.

Quite an unsavoury lot, they were now on board, primed and ready to offer illegal substances to young female passengers as they got ready for a 'fun-packed' night of drugs and debauchery.

The first evening on board began innocently enough. Dianne was enjoying herself immensely, drinking, dancing and socialising in the Legends Sports Bar with a number of adults, including her sister, Alma, and Gamu Chard, the son of some friends who were also travelling. With a few rum and cokes down her neck, she was in a festive mood, but as a lady who loved dancing, she found the music too light to really 'get down' and had to wait until 11 pm when the Starlight Disco opened with more exciting sounds. Around 9 pm, Alma left the dance floor to check on the children, Tahlia and Kari-Anne, and about an hour later Dianne also went back to their cabin to kiss her daughter goodnight and freshen up, saying to Nancy Chard, one of the group, 'See you later'.

Dianne and Gamu headed for the Starlight Disco when it opened, getting straight onto the dance floor, leaving their drinks on their table. Taking a break from time to time, they'd return to sit down, rest and order refills.

The alcohol clearly emboldened Dianne, as she approached several men for a dance, one of whom she'd met earlier at the bar, purchasing drinks. His name was Dragan Losic. He was a guy who stood out; a big fellow, about a hundred and ninety-three centimetres tall (six feet four inches), broad-shouldered and with a distinctive goatee beard. It was 1.51 am.

'How's your holiday going?' he asked,

'Fine,' Dianne replied, and they carried on chatting for several minutes, exchanging all the usual small talk about where they were from, family and friends etc.

After a while, Dragan said, 'Nice to meet you,' and took his drinks back to Petar Pantic, who was waiting at a nearby table.

By 2.30 am, the crowd had thinned out, leaving just a few of the more hardy passengers to carry on dancing and partying. Dianne and Gamu were sitting near some of the eight Adelaide men and started talking to them. Then, across the room, Dianne noticed a short man with thinning hair, Stephen Hart, who was working on board the ship as a magician. Their eyes met and Dianne smiled at him. He walked over to her, had a brief chat and then asked her for a dance. Gamu was now sitting by himself, and after a little while, he decided to call it a night and head back to his cabin.

Meanwhile, Stephen Hart had taken a break from dancing with Dianne to drink his beer. On swallowing it, he found to his disgust that someone had dropped a cigarette into the glass. He excused himself to Dianne and left the disco to go back to his cabin.

At 3.30 am, half an hour before the official closing time for the disco, Dianne approached a group containing some of the Adelaide men and asked Dragan if she could join them.

'No worries', he replied.

She then asked him if he'd like to dance with her. However, he declined, as he was talking to one of the ships' security guards, Olsen Va'aFusuaga (Mr V) about various matters. Dragan's close friend, Petar then piped up, 'Do you mind, this is a private conversation'.

Dianne didn't take any offence and stayed with the group. Later, Ryan Kuchel joined them, and she asked *him* for a dance. Unfortunately, he'd been drinking most of the night and refused her offer, saying he was too tired. He subsequently left the group and went off to bed.

Dragan later suggested to Mark Wilhelm, who was also with the group, that he should take Dianne for a dance, which he did. After their dance, the pair re-joined the group, and following a few playful advances towards Dragan, which met with Petar's obvious disapproval, Dianne turned her attentions back to Mark.

At about 4.20 am, they all decided it was time to leave and go back to their cabins. The three men, Dragan, Petar and Mark walked out the disco with Dianne, but the group split up with Dragan and Petar going one way and Dianne and Mark another. Down on the deck below, an intoxicated and staggering Dianne pulled Mark into the female toilets to give him oral sex, behaviour that was most unlike her, but Mark, who was aroused from the stimulation she gave him, felt uncomfortable about what she was doing, so he stopped her and took her back to his cabin, D182.

When they got there, it was dark and quiet, and the other three occupants seemed to be asleep, so they climbed onto Mark's top bunk and had consensual vaginal sex, with Mark ejaculating early as a consequence of the alcohol he'd consumed and possibly drugs in his system. Dianne was very unhappy with his performance, telling him he was a dud root and that it was the worst sex she'd had in a long time.

It then became apparent that not all the other occupants of the room were asleep, as Leo Silvestri offered Mark a Viagra tablet. Dianne climbed down from Mark's bunk and began giving oral sex to Leo, who was on the lower left bunk in the cabin. Mark decided to leave them to it, as the Viagra didn't appear to be working, and he left the cabin still naked, but for some unknown reason, he collected a life jacket on the way.

He went into cabin D156, occupied by Natasha McCann, Lisa Davis, Kelly Davis (Lisa's sister) and Tanya Power, where Dragan Losic, Petar Pantic and Ryan Kuchel were chatting to the young women. One of the men left the cabin and came back a few minutes later, holding a glass bottle with a clear liquid that had a pink tinge to it. He told the young women it was fantasy. In the meantime, Mark kept going in and out of the room. He eventually sobered up a little and returned to his own cabin, where he put on some boxer shorts. On returning once more, he and the other men each took a capful of the liquid. Ryan Kuchel passed out almost immediately (most likely because of the combination of the fantasy and the alcohol which was already in his system). The bottle was then offered to the young women, who wisely turned down the chance to imbibe.

Meanwhile, Charlie Kambouris had awoken up from his slumber in D178 and gone across the corridor to D182, looking for Dragan and Petar. There, he saw not only Dianne lying on the floor, but also that she had defecated herself. He then went to D156 and told them what he'd seen and said that Mark had to clean her up, as the whole cabin smelled.

By that time, sunlight was creeping through the portholes of the cabins. Dawn had broken.

Mark went back to his cabin, where he saw a naked Dianne lying on top of a blanket, on the floor, with faeces on her buttocks. He wiped her backside and felt for a pulse, finding only a faint one. He woke Leo, and with his assistance, they carried Dianne into the shower, where they tried to wake her. Unfortunately, the cold water didn't do the trick and mucilage had started coming out of her mouth. It didn't look good. They carried her back to the bedroom and laid her on the floor between the bunks. With Leo's assistance, Mark dressed her after attempting expired air resuscitation. A further problem then presented itself in that a number of people had started moving along the corridors, most likely to get breakfast. The situation was looking desperate.

Lisa Davis rang cabin D182 at 8.45 am and spoke to Mark, who replied that there was something going down and that he couldn't talk. Shortly afterwards, he called for medical assistance and a Code Alpha (medical emergency) call went out over the P.A. system for cabin D182. The medical staff arrived promptly led by a nurse, Donna Winter, who saw Dianne's cyanosed (blue colour) body which was unresponsive, not breathing and with no pulse. Her jeans were wet around the groin area, and it was thought that she was incontinent of urine, but on further examination, the wetness was found to be due to the shower she'd been given by Mark and Leo earlier. The rest of the medical team arrived and ushered Mark out of the cabin so they could commence attempts to resuscitate Dianne.

Unfortunately, they were unsuccessful, and her life was pronounced extinct at 9.03 am on 24 September; the official cause of death being recorded as 'cardiac arrest due to unknown causes'. However, the post-mortem and toxicology reports that would determine the real cause of death were yet to be done.

The death was reported to Marine Area Command, and they, in consultation with police commanders, crime agencies and various other bodies, including legal services and P & O Cruises, began an immediate enquiry. Senior Constable Erdinc 'Dinch' Ozen of the Marine Area Command investigative group contacted Mike Drake, the operations manager of the South Pacific at P&O to order cabin D182 and Dianne Brimble's cabin, D188, to be sealed off and a crime scene guard placed outside.

Marine Area Command was used to dealing with deaths aboard cruise ships and other marine vessels, but this one proved to be quite different, as following a conference with crime agencies, a number of cross territorial issues were revealed.

The cruise ship was about ninety nautical miles off the coast of New South Wales, with the next scheduled port of call being Noumea, New Caledonia, where it would arrive on 26 September, two days later. It was agreed that two investigators, a crime scene officer and a fingerprint officer would be flown to Noumea to meet the ship and begin their investigations. Forensic officers, including a pathologist, would only carry out the post-mortem on the body when it was returned to Sydney.

On 25 September, Acting Sergeant Victor Rulewski and Senior Constable Erdinc Ozen flew to Noumea to await the arrival of the cruise ship. The crime scene and fingerprint officers were due in the following day.

At 7.30 am on Thursday 26 September, Acting Sergeant Victor Rulewski and Senior Constable Erdinc Ozen met the *Pacific Sky* at the dock, making contact with

Captain le-Metre and the chief officers of New Caledonian Quarantine and Federal Police, together with the ship's captain, staff captain, chief of security and other staff members, including the ship's senior doctor, Dr Damien McAliskey, who considered Dianne's death suspicious because a tablet had been found near her body, suggesting she may have died from a drug overdose.

The detectives then met Alma Wood, Dianne's sister, who, after brief introductions, was taken to the medical centre of the ship, where she formally identified the deceased. Dianne's body was then released and sent back to Sydney, where it would undergo a post-mortem to determine her cause of death.

The police officers then took a statement from Alma in order to establish Dianne's movements up to and including 24 September. She said her sister had been in good spirits and had been a heavy social drinker, but hadn't been known to take drugs. She hadn't been depressed or had any major medical problems other than some respiratory problems, which included chest infections, sinus and asthma. Alma was then allowed to collect her passport and possessions from the cabin so she could fly back to Australia with the children.

Next to be interviewed were the 'eight persons of interest', beginning with Mark Wilhelm, via a portable ERISP (Electronically Recorded Interview of a Suspected Person). He gave two security incident reports, in which he didn't admit to drug usage, although on the second, he stated that he'd taken four ecstasy tablets on board, two of which he'd taken on the evening of 23 September, throwing the other two overboard after the incident. He emphatically denied supplying anyone with any drug.

Next up was Letterio 'Leo' Silvestri, who said he didn't want to be formally interviewed in relation to the matter, but eventually agreed to make a statement. He said he'd been intoxicated on the evening of 23 September and had taken three sleeping tablets, so he couldn't remember anything. However, he did recall seeing, in his words, 'an ugly fat black bitch' on his bunk, who he'd pushed off, onto the floor of the cabin. He denied supplying drugs to anyone.

Matthew Slade said he'd gone to sleep early that evening, as he'd had a few drinks and taken a sleeping tablet given to him by Leo Silvestri. When he'd woken up early the following morning, wanting to have a cigarette, he'd got out of bed and seen Mark Wilhelm and Leo Silvestri near the doorway of bathroom. He said their voices had sounded panicky.

Ryan Kuchel said he'd seen Mark Wilhelm having sex with Dianne Brimble, but had left shortly afterwards to speak to some people in the corridor. He'd later gone to cabin D156 (which he misidentified as D146), where he'd fallen asleep, waking up later that morning. It's probable he'd passed out from a combination of alcohol and a capful of fantasy (GHB).

In the meantime Senior Sergeant Newell from the fingerprint examination unit and Sergeant Cairnduff from the crime scene unit began their examination of cabin D182, but as the occupants had been allowed to enter cabins D182 and D178 and take their belongings, the crime scene had been severely compromised.

After Acting Sergeant Victor Rulewski and Senior Constable Erdinc Ozen concluded their interviews for the day, they reported back to their Sydney office before deciding to explore the ship and mingle with the passengers, thinking that people might be more willing to open up and talk them in a more informal environment. Just after 8 pm, they met up with the four young women, Lisa Davis, her sister Kellie, and their two friends, Tanya and Natasha, who were socialising in the Piano Lounge. Since Dianne's death they'd become nervous and, as they said later, they were very frightened after seeing the two men standing near the dance floor, 'glaring' at them.

Detective Senior Constable Ozen approached them. 'Which of you ladies would like to dance with me?'

Lisa volunteered, and during the waltz said, 'I think you need to speak with us girls'.

'Why?' Ozen asked. 'Which cabin are you in?'

'D156.'

When Lisa told him that various men had been going in and out of their cabin on the fateful morning, one naked save for a life jacket, Ozen agreed with her opening statement.

On 27 September, the remainder of the 'eight persons of interest', namely Dragan Losic, Luigi Vitale, Petar Pantic, and Sakaleros 'Charlie' Kambouris, were scheduled to be interviewed, but they refused without the presence of their lawyer and wouldn't even give a brief version of events.

However, the four young women from D156 were more forthcoming. They described the goings on during the night, including the activities of the men that came to their cabin. Of particular interest was the water bottle that contained a liquid with a pink tinge to it. The young women said they'd refused it when offered, and the men had left it in their cabin. A search was begun, but it wasn't to be found, although some exhibits were collected from the other cabins in question, including D182, and forwarded on to the appropriate laboratories for examination in the hope some tangible evidence might be gleaned from them.

While the crime scene had been compromised, as luck would have it, a valuable piece of evidence had inadvertently been saved. On the evening of 24 September, two days prior to the arrival of the Sydney detectives, a young boy of primary school age had been wandering in the lobby where the ship's purser's desk was located. He'd come across a rectangular purple plastic object, and not realising what it was, had handed it in to Michael Boulton, a junior purser. Thinking nothing more of it, Boulton had entered the object into a lost property register and placed it into a box in the lost property safe. The following morning, he'd been working with another junior assistant purser, Michael Edgeworth, who'd recognised the object as a 64MB Sony memory stick from a digital camera. Prior to that, the P & O staff had been briefed about the circumstances surrounding Dianne Brimble's death and advised to be vigilant about the men from Adelaide, so Edgeworth had deleted the entry from the register and inserted the memory stick into his camera to find out what was on it. He'd seen lots of photographs of people socialising on the ship. But more importantly, he'd recognised some of the members of the group of eight from Adelaide, so realising the information could be vital for those investigating Dianne's death, he'd handed the stick to a senior officer, Russell Walters, who gave it to the police several days later. In turn, they put it into an exhibit bag, for later examination by experts in Sydney.

In the meantime, Dragan Losic and Charlie Kambouris called around to the purser's desk to enquire about the missing memory stick, but there was no record of it in the register and it couldn't be found in the safe.

Back in Sydney, a police computer expert examined the 64MB memory stick and found forty-one JPEG files on it. They initially consisted of regular family snaps, but on probing further, he found records of a hundred and fifty-six deleted image files and twenty-six deleted video files. He was able to restore many of the deleted image files, including thirty files from 23 and 24 September, which were to provide information as to what had happened on the night in question. The video files, however, had been overwritten and could not be accessed.

Among the first batch of retrieved photos was one recorded at 12.18 pm on 23 September, which showed a group shot of the eight men from Adelaide outside the Sydney cruise ship terminal 8. However, the remaining twenty-two image files (depicting sexual acts and several shots of Dianne's prone body with faeces on her buttocks, with several disturbing close-ups) were recorded between 4.50 am and 6.32 am on Tuesday, 24 September, providing a graphic insight into the night of drugs and depravities which had led up to the tragedy. Consequently, they were of great help to the police investigation.

Nevertheless, it took about four years of interviews and investigations, coupled with numerous problems such as health issues with Senior Constable Erdinc Ozen, before a formal inquest into Dianne Brimble's death on the *Pacific Sky* cruise ship was finally implemented.

Her body arrived at the Glebe Department of Forensic Medicine on the morning of 27 September 2002. The ship's doctor, Dr Damian McAliskey, stated on his certificate that her cause of death was 'cardiac arrest due to an unknown cause', a standard statement to describe an unknown cause of death. He further added, 'The death was not due [to] a communicable or contagious disease, nor HIV related'.

The post-mortem was carried out by Dr Johan Duflou, at 10 am on 28 September. A number of minor injuries were observed on Dianne's body. There was suffusion (a widespread reddening) of her face, but no evidence of neck compression or other cause of obstruction of the airway. However, there was fluid accumulation in her lungs and all of her organs were reportedly congested. Such symptoms are typical of an over dosage of a central nervous system (CNS) depressant or a combination of CNS depressants.

That conclusion was borne out by the subsequent toxicology report, which revealed that a blood sample taken at post-mortem was found to contain: gamma-hydroxybutyrate (GHB) 210 milligrams per litre and alcohol 0.127 grams per 100 millilitres of blood. Dianne's stomach contents also contained GHB 6300 milligrams per litre and liver fluid GHB 120 milligrams per litre. That clearly indicated an overdose of GHB, which had been exacerbated by the alcohol already in her system from an evening of drinking.

The inquest finally got underway on Monday, 9 March 2006. It was conducted by the Senior Deputy State Coroner, Jacqueline Milledge, a former police prosecutor who had been working at the coroner's court for seven years and had seen her share of tragedies. Her assisting council was Mr Ron Hoenig, a criminal barrister who had previously carried out much of his work in the Supreme Court. He began his opening address by stating, 'Dianne Brimble was killed by some person or persons, by someone slipping her a lethal dose of a date-rape drug without her knowledge for the sole purpose of their own sexual gratification and the sexual assault and abuse of Mrs Brimble'.

He then outlined what the police knew about what had occurred on the *Pacific Sky* and the evidence provided by witnesses.

He concluded with, 'The evidence will clearly show that Mrs Brimble was killed. The evidence will clearly show that Mrs Brimble, a dedicated mother of children, who took her youngest child on a cruise, no doubt using her life savings, was preyed upon by some people after having had administered to her a substance that broke her will or interfered with any ability for her to say "yes" or "no". As a result she was subject to terrible degradation which no human being, let alone a female, should be subjected to. And the way in which somebody who themselves is a prude about their own body and covers themselves up to be found in the undignified way in which she was found is nothing short of absolutely reprehensible'.

After that opening address, further evidence was provided by family members and David Mitchell, Dianne's long-term partner and Tahlia's father, as to Dianne's modest, prudish nature.

Naturally, all of Australia's major newspapers ran the story the following day, and for the next three years, the story and people involved were rarely out of the news media.

I eventually became caught up in the inquest after issuing a statement regarding the amount of gamma hydroxybutyrate (GHB) and alcohol detected in Dianne's body at the post-mortem. I stated in part, after providing some background to the drug, the following: 'Ms Brimble's blood level was 210 milligrams per litre (along with alcohol at 0.127 grams per decilitre). Single doses of GHB (25mg/Kg) produce peak serum levels of 24 – 102 milligrams per litre. Doses of 50 mg/Kg produce peak levels of 48 – 124 milligrams per litre. Given Ms Brimble's weight of 86 kg then, it would appear she would have ingested over 7 grams (and possibly as high as ~18 grams) of GHB. Therefore, it would appear Ms Brimble either received more than one dose of GHB or that she received a rather large dose (probably, in her drink/s) prior to the disco closing, with the possibility of a further dose thereafter. This is supported by the elevated blood level of GHB and the fact that there was still some GHB present in her stomach contents'.

On Thursday, 16 November 2006, I attended Glebe Coroner's Court and was cross-examined regarding the effects of GHB. I described the drug, also known as fantasy and liquid ecstasy, as a 'colourless to pale pink, odourless, slightly salty tasting liquid freely soluble in water and thereby, can be readily added undetected, to drinks at parties and dances. It is a drug which is often used in cases of date rape'.

I was certain Dianne Brimble had had more than one dose and that she could have been topped up throughout the evening and early morning, an observation supported by her behaviour when she'd left the disco in the early morning, and I suggested that the first dose could have been taken in the ship's nightclub between three and four in the morning.

Mr Ron Hoenig, the assisting counsel, asked me what Dianne Brimble's chances of surviving such a dose had been.

I had no choice but to answer, 'I'm sorry to say, virtually none'.

That was due to the fact that she'd had *both* alcohol and GHB in her blood, and *both* at elevated levels. Furthermore, GHB had been present in her stomach contents, most likely from a more recent ingestion, and had provided a source of further absorption into her blood, thus sealing her fate.

I was called back to the inquest on 27 November, 2006 and subjected to a rigorous cross-examination by Mr John Sheahan, Senior Counsel, and P & O's senior barrister because my earlier testimony apparently had potential implications for P&O's liability, and the culpability of the 'eight persons of interest'.

Under cross-examination, I admitted my calculations had just been estimates and ballpark figures and the problem was that since then, a great deal of credence had been placed on them. For example, the figures I'd previously given regarding the range of how much GHB Dianne would have appeared to have ingested was based on GHB consumption and subsequent blood levels detected in the literature and from casework.

GHB exhibits nonlinear kinetics, such that in higher doses, it causes increases in absorption and elimination half-lives (the time it takes for a drug to drop to half its previous level) and the time to peak the blood concentration after consuming the drug orally (the usual mode of ingestion). In other words, it's not possible to carry out a back calculation like those done for alcohol intoxication.

I had merely sought to show that it had been more than likely that Dianne had received more than one dose of GHB (allegedly a capful from a water bottle). Given an average cap on a standard water bottle is about eight millilitres and GHB solution about fifty per cent (the alleged solution had a pink tinge), the dose provided by just one capful would have been about four grams and two capfuls about eight grams, which is well within the ballpark figure. However, street drugs are often of questionable purity.

Another expert, Dr David Caldicott, a specialist commissioned by Mark Wilhelm, told the inquest that it was possible Dianne had taken more than one dose of GHB, but that there was no way of knowing for sure.

Meanwhile, the police had been busy conducting a number of further investigations, including the recording of phone calls of the 'eight persons of interest'. They resulted in what became known as the 'The Brimble Tapes', providing valuable information to the inquest.

After sixty-six hearing days and seventeen months, the inquest finally reached a conclusion on the afternoon of 26 July 2007. NSW Deputy State Coroner Jacqueline Milledge ruled there was enough evidence to charge known persons over Dianne's death. She then spoke to the court, saying, 'I find that Dianne Elizabeth Brimble died on 24 September, 2002 in cabin D182 of the P&O cruise ship *Pacific Sky*. I am satisfied that the evidence before me is capable of satisfying a jury beyond reasonable doubt that known persons have committed an indictable offence and that there is a reasonable prospect that a jury would convict the known persons of an indictable offence in relation to the cause of death of Mrs Brimble. I therefore terminate this inquest pursuant to section nineteen of the Coroner's Act of 1980 and refer all the papers to the Director of Public Prosecutions (DPP)'.

However, the brief, being the full complement of papers and materials from the coroner, didn't arrive at the office of the DPP until 21 January 2008 – some six years after Dianne's lifeless body had been found in the cruise ship cabin.

The brief (a misnomer if ever there was) comprised seventeen boxes of statements and exhibits, each needing sorting, analysis and comment. Given the department was under resourced at the time, it was a lot to expect. However, after eight months of examining the evidence obtained from the coronial inquest, the DPP was able to make a recommendation that three of the four men who had shared cabin D182, where Dianne's body had been found, should face charges.

Mark Wilhelm should be charged with manslaughter and drug supply, for giving Dianne Brimble the drug GHB, while the other two men, Letterio 'Leo' Silvestri and Ryan Kuchel, should be charged with perverting the course of justice.

A statement was then issued from the DPP, announcing, 'Ex officio indictments for these charges have been filed in New South Wales with the district court regarding Silvestri and Kuchel and will be sought in the Supreme Court regarding Wilhelm'.

Mark Wilhelm's trial finally began in September 2009, seven years after Dianne Brimble's death. He appeared before Justice Roderick Howie at the Supreme Court, sitting in the Darlinghurst Court Complex at Taylor Square, Sydney. Justice Howie was an experienced appeal court judge who had presided over a number of high-profile cases over the years. The crown prosecutor was Mark Hobart, Senior Counsel, and the defence barrister was George Thomas.

I was subsequently subpoenaed to appear on 14 September, but that was complicated by the presence of myself and another three experts. The object of the exercise was to ascertain the extent of agreement and/or disagreement between the experts. A *voir dire* was held in the absence of the jury, in which we had to give joint evidence regarding the matter. A *voir dire* with *several* experts is seldom used in criminal matters, and it caught me by surprise. Fortunately, we agreed on most of the important issues, the exception being when Dianne had died. I felt that she'd been in serious trouble, if not already dying, when she'd defecated herself, as GHB can cause incontinence.

That latter piece of information was of importance in relation to a duty of care by Mark Wilhelm and Leo Silvestri, but it soon became apparent that the prosecution did not have a strong case for Wilhelm to be found guilty of manslaughter by negligence, leaving the remaining charge of drug supply.

The jury's deliberations dragged on, as there was uncertainty as to whether the drug had significantly caused Dianne's death and whether Wilhelm could be held criminally responsible. In the end, the jurors were unable to agree, resulting in a hung jury and another trial.

After the trial, Mark Wilhelm's lawyers offered the DPP a deal: if they dropped the manslaughter charge, he would plead guilty to the drug supply charge.

In the meantime, both the prosecution and defence teams searched the Crimes Act, and found a seldom used charge of using a noxious substance to endanger life.

On 29 April 2010, days before Mark Wilhelm's second trial was to go ahead, the DPP agreed, and withdrew the manslaughter charge. Later, Mark Wilhelm pleaded guilty to supplying Dianne Brimble with GHB.

Supreme Court Justice Howie described the supply of GHB as 'a "social" or consensual one, with the evidence showing both Mr Wilhelm and Ms Brimble took the drug willingly, as adults, ahead of a sexual encounter. Therefore on the scale of supply, it must be on the absolute lowest range of such offences'.

He then imposed a section 10, meaning no conviction was to be recorded.

He concluded, 'Finally it has come to an end and you can get on, hopefully, with the rest of your life the best as you are able'.

It was truly a sad end for an event that affected so many people, and all from a few drunken and drug affected hours.

On 5 March 2013, Detective Senior Constable Erdinc Ozen, a Turkish-born Australian, passed away from a brain aneurism. He was just forty-one years old. He'd previously retired from Marine Area Command on 29 September 2011, after completing twenty years of service. He'd been a fine dedicated police officer, and his colleagues, including myself, were greatly saddened by his passing. No doubt the stresses over the years since the death of Dianne Brimble and the subsequent inquest had taken their toll on his health.

The funeral service was held at Gelibolu Mosque, Gelibolu Avenue, Auburn on 8 March 2013, and unfortunately, this sad event was further marred by controversy when a Muslim cleric, Dr Abdurrahman Asaroglu, told everyone that because it was a Muslim prayer service, women and non-Muslims were not welcome and had to leave the mosque area. Erdinc's brother, Tunc Ozen said, 'All of his friends were not Muslim, so they had to leave. It was a big shock. It upset a lot of people'.

But probably, the most hurtful and upsetting thing for Erdinc's family came when it was time to move his coffin because his closest friends were not allowed to take part in the proceedings.

Tunc Ozen further commented, 'These complete strangers were grabbing my brother's coffin, not his mates, as a result of what this bloke said. I've spent as much time thanking people for coming as I have apologising to them over what happened'.

The Islamic Friendship Association president, Keysar Trad, said, 'What was done does not run consistently with our traditions. Our religion teaches us to be compassionate towards people grieving'.

For right or wrong, what was done was done and can't be undone, but it won't change people's opinion of Detective Senior Constable Erdinc Ozen, who will be remembered as a top cop who did his best, given the very difficult circumstances – and in the first case of its kind in Australia.

18

A Betrayal of Trust: The Peter Scott Case

'The worst pain in the world goes beyond the physical.
Even further beyond any other emotional pain
one can feel. It is the betrayal of a friend.'
~ Heather Brewer, *'Nine Grade Slays'*

Cromer is a suburb of northern Sydney, New South Wales. It's located twenty kilometres north-east of the Sydney central business district and bordered to the north by Narrabeen Lakes (also known as Narrabeen Lagoon). The area is administered by the local government area of Warringah Council and is part of the Northern Beaches region. For students, it's a delightful beachside suburb where they can get an education coupled with seaside sports, and for both adults and youngsters alike, it's a place for the ultimate in healthy lifestyles.

Peter Wayne Scott, or Scotty as he was affectionately known, was a talented, much loved teacher of visual arts at Cromer High. He was 'cool', prepared to bend the rules a little, understood the 'street cred' of his pupils and possessed an extraordinary talent for composing popular music. All in all, everything that made him a trusted and respected friend.

He began a successful local music business called B# Sharp Productions, which produced rock videos for bands such as the Divinyls, Mental as Anything and the Choirboys, receiving, in 1986, the prestigious Countdown Award for the best video. Some of his videos were also included in the 1986 Australian Art Perspecta and some major international galleries.

But behind that superficial veneer, there was something very sinister going on. In reality, he was a wolf in sheep's clothing.

Peter Scott was a man with homosexual yearnings, which is fine, only he crossed over to the dark side of his nature and began grooming, then drugging and sexually abusing teenage boys in his care. He assaulted boys in classrooms, in storerooms, during school hours or after school in his blue panel van emblazoned with the B # Sharp Productions logo.

One of his victims was regularly sexually assaulted two to three times a week. Scott would take him into a cleaner's room, give him a joint (of cannabis), pull his trousers down and perform fellatio on him. The student didn't dare move or say anything because he was too scared. In another instance, which occurred sometime between May and June 1985, Scott told one of his students that he would make a good model for one of his artworks - a mould or cast of the human body - because he didn't have much body hair, and asked him to stay after class. Scott took him to the school storeroom, which contained a kiln and was out of sight of other teachers and students, where he reiterated that the teenager would make a good model due to his lack of body hair and then subjected him to an embarrassing and unwanted examination of his private parts.

Saturday, 19 October 1985 was the day after the fifteenth birthday of another male student. That night, Scott drove him to a secluded car park at Jamison Park, Narrabeen. They were in the well-known van, which had tinted windows and a mattress in the rear parcel tray. Once settled, Scott supplied the teenager with a joint, allegedly sprinkled with heroin. When the youngster smoked the cigarette, he passed out almost immediately. On waking, he felt Scott was about to penetrate his anus with his erect penis. As he started to move away, a uniformed police officer came over and knocked on the window of the vehicle.

'What's going on?' Seeing the teenager, he asked him, 'Are you alright?'

The teenager, fearing he'd done something wrong, which he hadn't, said, 'I'm alright. This man is my uncle'.

Over time, the paedophile Scott lured many more teenage boys into various private places, plying them with heroin, cannabis and speed (methylamphetamine) before sexually assaulting them. As he moved on to further fields and other prey, he left behind victims who had not only been sexually abused, but who had also become addicted to the various substances administered to them during their sex sessions.

Scott's appalling behaviour continued for many years, in several other schools. He moved onto Mullumbimby High School, where he worked for a couple of years, and in 1989, when he chose the Byron Bay area as his new haven, the region's schools were unknowingly taking on a seasoned predator. He accepted a position as a visual arts teacher in 1989, at Bryon Bay High School, and taught there until 2010, quickly establishing himself as the top film technician in the area, working on many television commercials and documentaries. He worked in every area of the film industry, from sound, camera and editing, to directing and producing films for international broadcast. All the while, he kept his nefarious activities hidden.

It was only when some of his victims eventually plucked up the courage to come forward, some two decades after he'd started his reign of terror that he was eventually brought to account for some of his crimes. And that followed an intensive two-year investigation led by police from the Northern Beaches Local Area Command.

One day, in January 2012, he received an unexpected knock on his door in South Golden Beach, Byron Bay. A dishevelled Peter Scott was confronted by police bearing a warrant for his arrest. It contained charges of sexually assaulting three male students between 1984 and 1987 when he'd taught at Cromer High

School, on Sydney's Northern Beaches. There were a further nine charges to follow, including administering an intoxicating substance, committing an indictable offence, indecent assault and supplying a prohibited drug.

'Are you Peter Wayne Scott?' the police officer asked.

'Yes, I am', Scott replied. 'What's the problem?'

'We have a warrant for your arrest.'

Scott was taken to Byron Bay police station to prepare the first of several statements with regard to the charges. By the time he was arrested, Scott had spent just over forty years in the teaching profession, but had been shunted into an administration role at Byron High following the first complaints about his abuse by former Cromer High students.

The matter went before the Department of Public Prosecutions to determine if there was enough evidence to proceed to trial, with the evidence of the former three male students being deemed to be sufficient.

It was time for Scott to face the music, but certainly not in B Sharp!

It was to be a marathon trial, or rather, trials, involving five male students. Two separate trials were held at the Sydney Downing Centre District Court over four months, beginning in February 2013, and a further three trials took place from February 2014.

A media blackout was placed on each one and the victims' names were suppressed. Peter Scott, then aged sixty-two, faced charges of child sex and drug supply over a series of incidents at Cromer High School in the mid-1980s with teenage boys aged between fourteen and sixteen years of age.

It was a demanding time for all concerned, not just for the victims, but also for the individual witnesses, some of whom, including myself, attended the court on a number of occasions over the year. As for Scott, he continued with his administration duties at Byron Bay High School pending the outcome of the trials.

In her opening address to the jury, the crown prosecutor, Ms Nanette Williams, said that Scott had initially befriended his year eight students in various places, including the beach, where he took them to go surfing and gave them cannabis, telling them they weren't to let anybody know. Speaking about one of the unnamed students in particular, she said that Scott had 'started to have oral sex and masturbate him, and then masturbated himself. You will hear that this happened, on average, one or two times a week when the two were alone at school and that it happened for a long period of time, until the young man was in year ten'.

Ms Williams went on to say that one of these incidents had taken place in the second half of 1984, in the cleaner's room, which was above the school's gymnasium. 'The accused said he would give (the teenage boy) pot, and once there he made a joint. He then performed fellatio on him. The alleged victim will tell you that he froze and didn't want to move or say anything because he was too scared.' She also told the jury how while the offence was taking place the school's cleaner, Mr Lenny Taylor, had walked into the room, muttered something under his breath and promptly left.

Ms Williams described a number of other specific incidents, including the one of the boy on the night after his fifteenth birthday, who had been given cannabis laced with heroin by Scott, and had later found himself lying in the teacher's van with his trousers around his ankles.

However, Scott's defence barrister, Mr Matt Johnston, disputed the allegations against his client and doubted that the evidence of the alleged victim could be 'accepted as a witness of truth'.

One victim related to the court how the teacher had begun socialising with him and his friends during 1984 and 1985, in his first couple of years at Cromer High, and how he'd opened up the school's music room after hours and on weekends so they could have jam sessions. Scott would often give a joint to the teenage boys during those sessions, thus making them more vulnerable to the sexual abuse that followed.

Another victim recalled how on returning from a visit to the beach to go surfing with some of his friends, Scott had invited him back to his two-storey house at Bilgola so they could have a shower. The teacher had told him to use a shower upstairs while his friends had stayed downstairs. While in the shower,

Scott had joined him and indecently assaulted him.

Further evidence was given on Peter Scott's ability to groom the boys for his ends. Crown prosecutor Williams told the court, 'The accused, you might think, not only groomed the boys, but he groomed the school community. He groomed the family of [one victim]. Strong evidence came from his mother that she thought he was a good guy. He was somebody she welcomed into her house, she trusted him with her son. She trusted the accused with her son'.

I was at the trial to interpret the effects of the drugs that had been given to three of his teenage male victims, with particular attention being paid to the effects of heroin, methylamphetamine (speed), marijuana (cannabis) and cocaine.

In answer to questioning, I said:

> Heroin or diacetylmorphine is a potent opiate analgesic (pain reliever) which is rapidly broken down (half-life two to six minutes) to morphine. The pharmacology essentially then becomes that of morphine. Adverse or toxic effects of morphine usage include pinpointed pupils, nausea, drowsiness, dizziness, respiratory depression, constipation, hypotension (lowered blood pressure), pulmonary oedema and impairment of cognition and motor control.
>
> While methylamphetamine (also known as methylamphetamine, speed) and amphetamine are central nervous system (CNS) stimulants which can impair a user's faculties by altering perceptions and judgment and increase aggressive or risk-taking behaviour during the acute phase of intoxication, these drugs may also produce hallucinations. Following the stimulation phase, as the blood concentrations of the stimulants decrease, there may be a reactive drug-induced fatigue stage when a user's faculties can also be impaired. During this stage the user may experience drowsiness/sleepiness/fatigue, a slowing of reactions and impairment of perceptions and judgment.

> Cannabis or marijuana preparations are mainly derived from the female plant of Cannabis sativa. Delta-9-tetrahydrocannabinol (or delta-9-THC) is the major psychoactive active drug present in cannabis. Peak blood levels of delta-9-THC occur within minutes of smoking, and frequently the level drops to undetectable levels (by the procedures and analytical methods used in NSW) within one to two hours. However, impairment due to cannabis lasts some four to six hours after smoking. Delta-9-THC causes euphoria and relaxation, changes in memory, motor co-ordination, cognition, intensification of ordinary sensory experiences, and sense of time. When used in a social setting, the drug may produce talkativeness, hunger (the 'munchies') and infectious laughter.

I was further questioned about the effects of one of the victims having being supplied with speed or amphetamines at the age of thirteen years old and how it would affect someone of that age. The symptoms had been given by the victim, as he'd said, 'I talked a lot and it made me paranoid. I couldn't keep still in the gym. I was as high as a kite'.

I commented that that would appear to be consistent with the ingestion of a stimulant drug, for example, methylamphetamine or amphetamine.

In answer to the question, 'Would the complainant have been able to fend off an assault if under the influence of these drugs?' I replied, 'This depends upon the amount of drugs ingested by the victim and his tolerance to these drugs. However, if under the influence of heroin/morphine and cannabis, a person's ability to fend off possible unwanted sexual advances would be compromised. All of these drugs are CNS depressants'.

The question was explored further. 'The complainant had just turned fifteen years of age. Can you comment on the age of the complainant using these types of drugs?'

I pondered on this question for a short time before saying, 'Once a person of either sex reaches puberty, the pharmacokinetics for drug distribution is very similar to that of an adult. However, this does, of course, depend upon blood volume and subsequent distribution in the body of a person. Therefore, a small person would be more affected by a given dose of a drug than say, a large person. Other confounding factors include tolerance to a particular drug and various medical conditions. So, if the fifteen-year-old boy had little tolerance to these drugs (eg. cannabis, heroin, amphetamines) and was of a lesser body weight than an experienced adult, then he would be expected to more greatly affected'.

A further question followed. 'Are you able to comment on the stated feelings of the complainant about feeling high and anxious?'

I replied, 'Cannabis (marijuana) affects almost every part of the body. It combines many of the properties of alcohol, tranquillisers and hallucinogens; it is a sedative, analgesic and anxiolytic. It stimulates the appetite and has many systemic effects. Therefore, a person would possibly experience a high (drug affected) but feelings of being anxious would most likely be attributed to the circumstances the young person found himself in as the anxiolytic effects of the drug wore off'.

The defence then asked if marijuana had been a stupefying drug in 1985. It was a question I found quite amazing, but maybe it related to the legislation in force at the time he was focusing on.

My answer was, 'Marijuana (cannabis) has always been a stupefying drug and central nervous depressant'.

Yet more questions were raised in relation to the matter.

'Is [are] cannabis, amphetamines and heroin drugs of addiction?'

I replied, 'Heroin is a powerful drug of addiction, amphetamines are not considered drugs of addiction, but a heavy user may become physically dependent upon the drug. The latter comment could also apply to cannabis'.

'Are cocaine and heroin stupefying drugs?'

'Cocaine is a CNS stimulant, whilst heroin is a CNS depressant. A stupefying drug is one that produces narcosis or stupor. Heroin would fall in to that category and the effects would be enhanced in the presence of cannabis.'

The court was told that Scott's offences had taken place at various locations, including Cromer High School, his Bilgola home and Jamieson Park at Narrabeen Lakes. The victims had been aged between eleven and fifteen at the time, and they gave victim impact statements to the court.

One victim of Scott's abuse told the court that he'd become addicted to heroin after leaving Cromer High School, saying, 'From time to time, I would go back to my family and try to clean up, but this was to no avail. I always ended up back on the streets'. Looking over to Peter Scott in the dock, he said, 'I became more and more aggressive towards others as I was frustrated from being abused by you so many times for so many years'. Then he paused in reflection before commenting, 'You will not be known as Scotty as we called you. You will be known as Peter Wayne Scott – paedophile'.

Scott denied all the allegations against him, even describing one of his victims as a nightmare, a thief and an aggressive stalker. Further, to his victim's dismay, he denied even knowing three of them (the final number will probably never be known), telling the court, 'I don't remember those students. I don't know them. I have no recall of them'.

The final betrayal by 'Mr Cool'.

On 2 May 2014, after a trial lasting a number of weeks, the jury found Scott guilty of fourteen charges relating to sexual assault offences against the five male students between 1984 and 1986, by a majority verdict.

At the sentencing hearing, Justice Sarah Huggett said, 'These acts were carried out by a teacher who adults trusted and who students thought was "cool" and nice. He is appropriately described as a sexual predator'.

In consideration of the sentence, she added, 'The offender was a married, mature man in his thirties, and I'm satisfied he committed each offence for his own sexual gratification'.

She then handed down the maximum sentence of fourteen years jail, with a non-parole period of seven and a half years. She also found that a number of the offences had been committed with a degree of planning and premeditation, and considered that a number of the offences were in the most serious category. Furthermore, she noted that the sentencing rules in place at the time of the offending, which she was required to abide by, showed greater leniency to offenders than the current laws, which meant for a lesser sentence than she could have given if the offences had been carried out in 2014.

Allowing for the time already spent in custody, Scott will be eligible for parole in September 2021.

19

The Justins and Jenning Case: Euthanasia or Murder?

'If Alzheimer's disease destroyed only unhappy memories – would we search for a cure?'

~ ***Anon***

Gaius Plinius Secundus, better known as Pliny the Elder, was a Roman author, naturalist and natural philosopher as well as a naval and army commander of the early Roman Empire (23 AD). He once said, *'Only a physician can commit homicide with impunity'*. Dr Harold Shipman (a proven serial murderer), for one, would not have disagreed with him!

The issue of euthanasia has always been a subject of much controversy, and over time, it's taken on some bizarre twists, for example, the development of a 'suicide machine' by Dr Philip Nitschke in the Northern Territory, Australia.

The device involved a computer that asked the patient three times whether they really wanted to die. If the patient answered in the affirmative, on each response, a hundred millilitres of liquid Nembutal was pumped into their arm. They also received 6.39 grams of sodium pentobarbitone, causing them to fall asleep and die within minutes. Then there are a number of self-help books, notably Derek Humphrey's *Final Exit,* originally published in 1997, which became a best seller, and more recently, Dr Nitschke's publication, *Killing Me Softly: Voluntary Euthanasia and the Road to the Peaceful Pill,* about how to commit suicide.

Those developments came about due to a growing public wariness of the health care system, which uses advanced life support systems to prolong the lives of dying patients, often against the wishes of them and their relatives.

Because of the seemingly unnecessary prolongation of very sick, seriously infirm and terminal patients, a movement has grown for so-called passive euthanasia, and medical ethicists and members of the public alike accept that a mentally competent adult who is in severe chronic pain or who is terminally ill has the right to choose to be removed from a ventilator and/or drip feeding – a view which the courts have so far upheld.

However, the problem is active euthanasia, in which a patient's life is ended intentionally and directly, for example, by means of a lethal injection. Many supporters of active euthanasia, including Exit International, believe that it should be made legal for patients who have made a rational decision to end their lives and thus reduce pain and suffering. But opponents of active euthanasia fear it may lead to doctors and health care personnel being cast in the role of takers of life, rather than savers of life, which is a distinct conflict of interest for doctors who follow the Hippocratic Oath.

But is there any difference between stopping a patient's life support and administering a lethal injection, if both acts lead to a patient's death? Administering a lethal dosage of a drug and stopping life support are, morally speaking, the same, given the same outcome.

What really matters are the person's intentions for acting (or not acting).

As for the actual carrying out of the deed, Nembutal, one of several trade names for the drug sodium pentobarbitone (or sodium pentobarbital as it is known in the USA), is the favoured drug of choice for both animals and humans. It's used in Switzerland, Belgium, Netherlands and Oregon, USA, as part of their legal euthanasia programs. Exit International, the non-profit Australian public company, have identified a number of overseas places where it's possible to obtain the drug over the counter, one of them being Mexico, where sterile Nembutal is readily available from veterinary supply shops. It comes in a sealed bottle and is undetectable by airport X-ray equipment.

Exit International is one of a small number of assisted suicide organisations that includes Dignitas and Final EXIT. Founded in 1997 by Dr Philip Nitschke, its website says it has twenty thousand online members around the world.

It was about 8.30 am on 22 March, 2006 when seventy-one-year-old former Qantas airline pilot Graeme William Wylie sat down on his favourite sofa in the living room of his two-storey home at Cammeray to enjoy a very humble breakfast of toast and a mug of hot water. It had been served up a short while earlier by his de-facto of eighteen years, fifty-eight-year-old Shirley Justins. Having performed her domestic duty, she left the house and drove to Kensington before going on to Marrickville, where she went shopping with a friend. When she returned at about midday, Wylie appeared to still be sitting in a relaxed position in the living room. Only he wasn't – he was dead.

Five hours later, Shirley notified the police. When they arrived, she told them that Wylie had had a lengthy history of Alzheimer's disease and had been taking medication for the condition.

There was a newspaper near his body, open at an article highlighted in biro. It was entitled: 'Study of Alzheimer's Drug Revives Questions on Risk'. The article described the drug Aricept, which is used to treat people suffering from Alzheimer's, but more importantly, part of it had been bracketed in biro. It read: 'An unusual number of deaths among patients in a large study of Aricept, the most popular drug to treat Alzheimer's disease, is raising concern among federal officials and some disease experts. Judee Shuler, an Eisai spokeswoman said the study results were a statistical fluke. Patients given placebos in the study were unusually healthy, she said, making a comparison with the group taking Aricept unfair. Aricept remains safe, Ms Shuler said, and the company is not recommending any changes to the drug's label'.

A comment, written in biro, with an arrow directed from that paragraph, said: 'In support of her company, she would say this!'

Rigor mortis in the body indicated that Wylie's death had occurred a few hours earlier. He was subsequently declared deceased and his body taken away for a post-mortem examination.

A blood sample taken at the autopsy was found to contain the following:

- pentobarbitone 22.0 milligrams per litre,
- metoclopramide 0.8 milligrams per litre,
- paracetamol less than 3.0 milligrams per litre, and
- alcohol 0.007 grams (100 millilitres) of blood. No donepezil (Aricept) was detected.

The small amount of paracetamol was probably derived from a Panadol or Panamax tablet Wylie had consumed sometime earlier, while the trace amount of alcohol could have been a residual level left over from a previous evening's drink. However, the levels of metoclopramide and pentobarbitone were particularly significant. The presence of metoclopramide in Wylie's blood was no surprise as it had been prescribed as Maxolon (10 mg tablets) by his local doctor at the Chatswood Medical Centre. Metoclopramide (Maxolon) is used to treat nausea and vomiting, which are unfortunate side-effects of donepezil (Aricept) therapy and other opiate drugs, such as oxycodone, and it's also been used to prevent and treat irradiation sickness, post-operative vomiting and drug induced nausea. So while its presence was not a surprise, the level of it was.

The usual therapeutic range for metoclopramide in the blood is from 0.07 to 0.13 milligrams per litre of blood. Wylie's blood level for metoclopramide was 0.8 mg/L, which was just over six times the upper level.

As for the pentobarbitone, that had not been prescribed to Wylie.

I formed the opinion that the blood concentration of pentobarbitone, together with a compromised respiratory condition (lung infection), would have led to his death, and that the elevated level of metoclopramide may have exacerbated those conditions.

The drug is a short-acting barbiturate that has been applied as a hypnotic in the treatment of insomnia as well as a sedative. It's also been used as a basal narcotic prior to the administration of an inhalation anaesthetic. For that purpose, 100 to 200 milligrams may be given orally to the patient prior to an operation. Veterinary practices are equally known to have employed it to euthanize very sick and dying animals, and it's available under the very descriptive trade name of Lethabarb.

The usual therapeutic range for pentobarbitone in the blood ranges from 1 - 4 mg/L. Graeme Wylie's blood level was 22 mg/L, which is just over five and a half times the upper level and well within the toxic range, certainly lethal for a novice user.

In October 2002, following six years of cognitive decline, Wylie had been referred to the cognitive disorders clinic at Concord Hospital by Dr Kujan Nagaratnam. The diagnosis had been a wasting of the mental faculties of a very intelligent man who had been a skilled and capable pilot. He'd been further assessed in March 2003 by Ms Therese Alting, a clinical neuropsychologist, who had determined that he'd had a wide range of cognitive impairments, including language, visual-spiral, attentional, executive and memory skills; and that the impairments, which had been apparent across the spectrum of cognitive domains, together with Wylie's gradual cognitive decline, had been consistent with Alzheimer's disease.

At the cognitive disorders clinic, Wylie had initially been under the care of Dr Valerie Fletcher, who had reported that the disease had been developing in him since his late fifties, shortly after he'd retired from Qantas as an airline pilot. In August 2003, Dr John Cullen had begun reviewing and assessing Wylie's Alzheimer's disease at regular six-month intervals. In his most recent assessment, in August 2005, he had been prescribed Aricept by his general practitioner, Dr Russell, to treat his Alzheimer's, which he'd continued to take on a daily basis.

Six months later, on 2 February 2006, Wylie had fallen over and wound up in the Royal North Shore Hospital for two weeks, where he'd been treated for fractures to the top of his left leg and right shoulder. He'd been discharged on 20 February and prescribed a number of medications including Endone (oxycodone) to ease his pain. However, just three days after his discharge, both he and Shirley Justins had visited the Chatswood Medical Centre for treatment of his pain and nausea, where Dr Gupta had wisely advised Graeme to stop taking the Endone, which had probably been causing some of his nausea. He'd then been prescribed Maxolon 10mg tablets (a brand of metoclopramide) to treat his nausea and Ostelin Vitamin D capsules to help strengthen his bones.

Graeme Wylie had clearly been in the advanced stages of Alzheimer's disease.

Prior to that, Shirley Justins and her friend, seventy-three-year-old Caren Jenning, had failed in an application for assisted suicide (active euthanasia) to the Swiss organisation Dignitas because Wylie had been considered unable to make a rational decision to end his life. Perhaps there was another way.

Caren Jenning had been diagnosed with breast cancer and the disease had moved to other parts of her body. The prognosis wasn't good, and as a long time active member of Exit International, she'd also been exploring ways of ending her own life. She had the motivation as well as the means, and no doubt had imparted such information to Shirley Justins as a possible way of dealing with her situation.

After the results of Graeme Wylie's post-mortem and toxicology results were released, police investigators swung into action. They obtained a search warrant for Caren Jenning's residence, and among various items, they found a Quill black notebook labelled EXIT, inside which was a page entitled Practical Workshop Handbook, which contained the following notes in Shirley Justins' hand:

10 grams of liquid Nembutal

Fly to Mexico! Or Lethabarb

ANESTESAL in Mexico, Tijuana Vet supply shops

N.B. Stemetil or Maxilon [sic] to inhibit vomiting for 2 previous days, 2 tablets every 2 hours.

Some tea and toast so stomach not empty.

Also included were alternative drug combinations such Doloxene (a preparation containing dextropropoxyphene) and Serapax (oxazepam):

100 capsules, opened & powder stirred into a drink – it doesn't dissolve.

But fortunately, she also included:

Avoid paracetamol (ie DI-GESIC) or Panadeine – yes death, but nasty!

Di-Gesic is a preparation containing both paracetamol and dextropropoxyphene, a very effective combination for pain relief. Excessive amounts of paracetamol severely damage the liver, while products containing dextropropoxyphene have been associated with cardiac conduction abnormalities that may lead to life threatening arrhythmias. They aren't recommended for older people and those with a known history of cardiovascular disease, decreased kidney function or a history of depression or mental illness. There are only two dextropropoxyphene-containing analgesics registered in Australia: Di-Gesic and Doloxene.

Wisely, Shirley avoided those drug combinations. Her drug of choice was Nembutal, or the Mexican version, Anestesal, which are just different trade names for the same drug, pentobarbitone or pentobarbital, the peaceful, painless death drug.

The investigators had found a recipe book for death.

On Sunday, 25 February 2007, Shirley Justins and Caren Jenning were charged with murdering Graeme Wylie with a lethal drug overdose. Caren Jenning was arrested at her Lane Cove retirement village, and both she and Shirley Justins were taken to cells at the Sydney Police Centre, as no room was available at Mulawa women's prison. Their arrests followed an eleven-month investigation by detectives from north Sydney police and homicide investigators attached to the coroner's investigation unit.

It was an unusual case, as they were believed to be the first murder charges linked to an alleged mercy killing in New South Wales.

The matter initially went before the Manly Local Court on Tuesday, 27 February 2007, where the two women appeared wearing handcuffs. They were formally charged with murdering Graeme Wylie with Nembutal, a barbiturate not sold in Australia for human use. The prosecution alleged that Wylie's dementia had been such that he'd been incapable of searching for the drug in Australia and that he hadn't travelled to Mexico, the only country where the drug can be purchased, though it was probable that Caren Jenning had been aware of that when she'd travelled to Tijuana in mid-March, 2006.

The defence barrister, Mr Paul Glissan, said that Shirley Justins, a National Trust bush regenerator, had no connection with Mr Wylie's death, but the prosecution then alleged that not only had various listening devices recorded her talking about Nembutal, but they also had the Quill black notebook labelled EXIT, containing the Practical Workshop Handbook notes.

Both women applied for bail, claiming exceptional circumstances; Caren Jenning due to her advanced cancer, which had travelled to her sternum and hip and required treatment, and Shirley Justins because she needed to travel to western Australia to tend to her sick mother, who was due to undergo surgery. Bail was refused and both women were remanded to appear in the Central Local Court on 6 March 2007.

Outside the court, Mr Glissan continued to maintain Shirley Justins' innocence, saying Graeme Wylie had long desired to end his life and that his client didn't know how the drug had come into his possession. After a week in custody, the two women were granted bail in the Central Local Court by Magistrate Paul Lyons after the Department of Public Prosecutions (DPP) said it would not oppose a bail application. Mr Geoff Denman, a DPP solicitor, told the court that the Crown conceded that the circumstances of both women were exceptional and agreed for them to be set free, pending the outcome of the case. Shirley Justins was granted one hundred and sixty thousand dollars bail, of which she had to deposit eighty thousand dollars as a surety, whilst Caren

Jenning was granted bail after three people said they would each provide a surety of ten thousand dollars. The matter then went before the NSW Supreme Court, being set down for 5 May 2008.

This case appeared before Justice Roderick Howie. Shirley Justins pleaded not guilty to murdering Graeme Wylie, her partner of eighteen years, and Caren Jenning pleaded not guilty to being an accessory before the fact. She also pleaded not guilty to importing the drug Nembutal into Australia. They both pleaded not guilty to the lesser alternative charge of aiding and abetting a suicide.

Crown prosecutor, Mr Mark Tedeschi, QC, opened with:

> The accused, Shirley Justins, had a strong financial motive to bring about his death and also a personal motive in wanting Mr Wylie deceased.
>
> Caren Jenning was ideologically motivated to assist Shirley Justins in bringing about the death of Graeme Wylie. She had a personal motive.
>
> If Mr Wylie was deemed to be mentally incapable of deciding to commit suicide, then providing him with the means to do so was murder – irrespective of the accused's reasons.
>
> Mr Wylie's mental health had deteriorated drastically in the ten years preceding his death. Mr Wylie was unable to manage his medication or financial affairs and could not (even) name his children. He was in a mentally befuddled condition and in no position to decide to take his own life. If Graeme Wylie was affected by dementia to the extent that he no longer had the capacity to make an independent, informed decision about whether or not to commit suicide, then from the law's point of view, it is though he did not know that the poison was there. These actions in taking Nembutal to him amount to murder. A decision made by a vulnerable,

incapacitated, sick person under the overwhelming influence or manipulation of another is no decision at all.

The court heard that two months before Graeme Wiley died from a barbiturate overdose he'd told a friend, 'My brain is fucked. I'm going to top myself before it's going to get any worse and while I still know what's going on'.

Shirley Justins told the court that he'd been, 'a proud, irascible man, who wanted a peaceful and dignified death. His life had become boring and he was unable to do what he enjoyed'.

Defence counsel, Mr Peter Bodor, QC, reiterated, 'He wanted to leave the world. He'd had enough'.

The court heard that there had been times when Mr Wylie had been totally with it and other times when he hadn't. In his lucid moments he'd also discussed suicide with his sisters. Peter Bodor also said, 'A week before his death he decided to get his affairs in order and changed his will'.

The crown prosecutor brought the court's attention to the fact that in the will, Shirley Justins stood to gain all but two hundred thousand dollars of Graeme Wylie's estate, valued at close on two and a half million dollars. Therefore, he reasoned, she had a motive to kill him, and had done so not out of loving kindness, but out of self-interest.

A general practitioner who had seen Wylie on several occasions before his death provided a certificate saying that he'd still been capable of making his own decisions and that he'd understood the nature of his decisions.

Mr Tedeschi, QC, responded by saying that the doctor had failed to make sufficient inquiries into Wylie's health. He also brought up the fact that Dignitas, the Swiss euthanasia organisation, had previously rejected Wylie's application for assisted death, as they'd considered him to be unable to make a rational decision to end his life due to his deteriorating mental condition. It therefore followed, he argued, that Shirley Justins and Caren Jenning had known Graeme Wylie had not been capable of making the decision to end his life.

Wylie's youngest daughter from a previous marriage, Mrs Nicola Dumbrell, took to the stand and told the jury that Caren Jenning had come to her house in December 2005 to explain the Dignitas application. She said her husband had asked her to come and explain how the application would proceed, given that Dignitas did not accept Alzheimer's patients.

Prior to Nicola Dumbrell taking the stand, the court had previously been told that Shirley Justins and Caren Jenning were members of Exit International and had consulted the director, Dr Phillip Nitschke, about their plans for Mr Wylie. Nembutal was the drug of choice of the organisation, and the jury were further informed of the notes found in Shirley Justins' handwriting about the use of the drug.

Mrs Dumbrell went on to explain that she and her husband had known very well that it was Caren who'd been instigating the whole thing.

Shirley Justins' barrister, Peter Bodor, QC, suggested that Nicola had constantly badgered Caren about her father's will after the Dignitas application had been sent off, but Nicola replied that she'd never asked to see the will, and that it hadn't been a matter of what she'd wanted, it had been a matter of getting the old wills and seeing what was available.

She said it had been the timing of the new will, drawn up a week before her father's death, which had concerned her, rather than its contents.

'I was unhappy with the date of the will. It was quite different from what I had been told three to four months earlier, when it had been a fair and equal will at that point.'

She added that she hadn't found out about the new will until after her father's death.

When questioned about the events of the fateful morning, Shirley Justins admitted she'd prepared a cup of water with a slice of lemon and opened a bottle of Nembutal, which she'd placed next to a glass on the table, saying to Wylie, 'This will relieve your pain, Graeme. If you drink this you will die'. Wylie had apparently said, 'Yes' before pouring the drug into the glass and drinking the contents, allegedly losing consciousness almost immediately. After that, Shirley Justins had left the house, returning later in the day to find that he'd died.

She pleaded guilty to aiding and abetting Graeme Wylie's suicide, while Caren Jenning pleaded guilty to importing the border–controlled drug Nembutal.

However, they both pleaded not guilty to the more serious charges of murder and of being an accessory before the crime.

The crown prosecutor rejected the lesser guilty pleas, insisting that the more serious charges of murder and being an accessory should stand.

Justice Roderick Howie told the jury that they needed to consider whether Shirley Justins' actions had constituted murder and whether Caren Jenning had been an accessory to the offence. He addressed the jury, saying, 'In the case of Shirley Justins, the situation is that the trial is proceeding in relation to the charge of murder. It is also proceeding on the lesser charge of aiding and abetting suicide. However, you can take into account her plea of guilty as, in effect, an admission of that offence. It would be expected that if you find her not guilty of murder you will find her guilty of being an accessory before the fact of murder, or aiding and abetting suicide'.

In Caren Jenning's case, he said that it was still open to the jury to find her guilty of being an accessory before the fact of murder, or aiding and abetting suicide, but the separate charge of importing Nembutal was no longer before them.

The controversial euthanasia advocate, Dr Phillip Nitschke, was called to testify on behalf of both Shirley Justins and Caren Jenning. He told the court that he'd assessed Graeme Wylie on behalf of Dignitas on 16 November, 2005, and prepared a report stating that Wylie 'appeared physically fit, despite ongoing unexplained dizziness (but was) able to travel to Switzerland. Graeme is significantly affected by dementia and depends a great deal on his carer, Shirley Justins. He was unable to recall his date of birth or number and sex of his children. He retains significant insight though, and realisation that his mental capacity is failing and it is causing him a great deal of distress. He (Graeme Wylie) is adamant he wants to go to Switzerland as soon as possible'.

Dr Nitschke appeared confident in his belief that Wylie had been capable of deciding on his assisted suicide, but disagreed that he (Dr Nitschke) had been ideologically driven.

The crown prosecutor put it to him thusly: 'You were hell bent on supporting Graeme Wylie's application to Dignitas, no matter what his condition, because of your ideological views on suicide'.

Dr Nitschke replied, 'That is incorrect, and I object to the term "hell bent"'.

The court was informed that Dr Nitschke had spoken to Graeme Wylie and Shirley Justins for two hours, but hadn't taken any notes, nor conducted any standardised cognitive tests, and had overlooked a number of specialist reports from Concord Hospital, where Wylie had been a patient for some years. Justice Roderick Howie asked Dr Nitschke if it would have been better to have gotten an independent doctor to assess Graeme Wylie to determine if he had been capable of making the decision to end his life, to which he replied, 'With the clarity of hindsight that is true, sir'.

The crown prosecutor said, 'You were negligent and careless in failing to ask to see any of [Mr Wylie's] medical reports'.

Dr Nitschke answered that he'd been there and the crown prosecutor hadn't. Furthermore, he'd had nothing to gain from supporting his application. He'd seen a frail man, a dying man, a suffering man, who had wanted help to die and anyone would have approved it.

The trial centred on Graeme Wylie's mental capabilities, with the prosecution arguing that his dementia had left him incapable of making an informed, independent choice to end his life. The crown prosecutor, Mark Tedeschi, pointed out that, 'If he (Graeme Wylie) lacked the capacity, (then) it was not suicide and the accused (Shirley Justins) put to death a very sick, feeble, confused and dependent old man'.

After six weeks, with three further days of deliberations, the jury, by a majority verdict, found Shirley Justins guilty of manslaughter rather than murder, finding that she had neglected her duty of care towards Graeme Wylie. Caren Jenning was found guilty of being an accessory before the fact to manslaughter, while the alternative charge of assisted suicide and the possibility that Graeme Wylie had been able to decide to end his life was rejected.

Neither woman showed any emotion as the verdicts were handed down, which was in direct contrast to their families and supporters, some of whom openly wept.

Outside the court, Nicola Dumbrell commented, 'I think the verdict is correct', while her sister, Ms Tania Shakespeare said, 'They broke the law. He (Graeme Wylie) didn't think of killing himself. He was always looking for a cure, he was never looking to die'.

However, the outcome was a disappointment for Dr Nitschke. He said he thought that, 'Mr Wylie still knew what he was doing', and further, that people with Alzheimer's and dementia, 'would have to end their lives before their time to ensure those helping them did not face murder charges'. He vowed to change the way his organisation Exit International advised people with similar problems in the future.

It was a complicated case, and some evidence was kept from the jury, which may, or may not, have changed the verdict reached. While the jurors were told about Shirley Justins' alleged financial motive, they were not told about her female lover, Bergi Mueller, in Germany, and the fact that police hadn't seen any female clothing or toiletries in Graeme Wylie's home at Cammeray, suggesting that he and Shirley Justins had no longer been in a committed relationship.

They were also not privy to Dr Nitschke's involvement in the suicide of Mrs Nancy Crick, who'd thought she had terminal cancer, but had, in fact, only had a readily treatable twisted bowel. A post-mortem report had shown no evidence of bowel cancer at the time she'd consumed a lethal dose of barbiturate. Furthermore, Dr Nitschke had only consented to give evidence after being subpoenaed and receiving a certificate against incrimination regarding questions into the activities of Exit International.

After the verdict, it was up to Justice Roderick Howie to deliver sentencing. Apart from the intricacies of the case, the matter was further complicated by the advanced ages of the two offenders. Given the severity of the women's crimes, Justice Howie could have imposed prison terms up to twenty-five years each, effectively sentencing them to die in gaol. However, that didn't eventuate, as manslaughter was the only indictment put before the jury and it wasn't to be a referendum on euthanasia.

The sentencing hearing was set for 7 October 2008.

The lawyers appearing for Caren Jenning indicated their intentions of seeking a non-custodial sentence due to what they termed the 'unusual circumstances of the case', but there was a further twist to come.

Both women potentially faced lengthy terms of imprisonment, but Caren Jenning, with her terminal breast cancer which had spread to the rest of her body, was not prepared to take the chance of being sent to prison. She'd kept some of her Mexican Nembutal (Anestesal) for herself, thinking that in her condition she may well have need of it in the future, and on Thursday night, 17 September, 2008, she consumed a lethal dose of the drug. She died peacefully and alone in her home at Lane Cove on the north shore of Sydney.

Before doing so, she mentioned her intentions to her daughter, Kate, and Dr Philip Nitschke, stating, 'I'm not going to die in jail, so I'm going to take a pre-emptive step'.

Kate said:

> My mother believed that everybody should have a choice. She was not a criminal deserving of a prison cell. Anyone like my mother who did what she did for Graeme Wylie out of compassion and respect should not be treated like one.
>
> By taking her own life it should not be said that she was running away from punishment. She was dying, she was in pain, and just could not bear the thought of living with that pain in jail. I share her views. I support her fully in what she did and I am proud of her. I am proud of what she has done so bravely.

A former judge, QC, and former head of the NSW Voluntary Euthanasia Society, Mr Keppel Earl 'Kep' Enderby, was shocked by her death, but said, 'She was one of the finest people I've ever known'.

The matter now appeared to have moved on from the issue of illegally taking a person's life to one on the merits of euthanasia, muddying Justice Howie's waters even further.

On the morning of 12 November 2008, in the NSW Supreme Court, he commenced his judgement. He was critical of some members of the community for turning the case into a forum about euthanasia. 'It [the case] has been seen by some members of the community as a test case for euthanasia or the right of someone to take their own life. It was no such thing. The law holds human life so sacred that it does not give permission for someone else to take it.'

He further added that Shirley Justins and Caren Jenning had acted in 'a joint criminal enterprise to bring about the death of the deceased,' before denouncing the killing by saying,

'A calculated and unlawful taking of human life is an affront to every aspect of civilised society.'

Justice Howie said Caren Jenning had been the driving force in the euthanasia plan, labelling the deceased woman as 'manipulative and dishonest' and, therefore, more criminally liable. He also mentioned that Graeme Wylie's two daughters had not had the opportunity to say their goodbyes to their father.

In the interest of deterrence, Justice Howie said it was necessary to give Shirley Justins a custodial sentence, as many in the community would have seen her conviction 'as a badge of honour rather than a mark of the community's disapproval'. He sentenced her to twenty-two months of periodic detention, to be released on parole on 20 September 2010.

Caren Jenning was to have been sentenced to a non-parole period of twenty-two months, with a balance of term of eight months, to be served by way of periodic detention.

Outside the court, Kate Jenning would not accept Justice Howie's finding that her mother had been involved in criminal activity. 'To be portrayed as a criminal and mastermind is abominable.'

Dr Nitschke praised the 'lenient sentence', but still maintained that Graeme Wylie had known he'd wanted to end his life, a view not shared by his daughters. Tania Shakespeare said her father hadn't been happy to have Alzheimer's disease, but he hadn't wanted to die. 'He needed better treatment and care.'

Just under two years later, after Shirley Justins had served her sentence, the Court of Criminal Appeal, consisting of Chief Justice Jim Spigelman, Justice Carolyn Simpson and Justice Peter Johnson heard the various arguments about the legal directions given by the trial judge, Justice Roderick Howie. Justice Simpson said the manslaughter charge should never have been allowed at the trial, as the prosecution had been insistent that the more serious charges of murder and being an accessory should have stood.

The tribunal considered questions of whether the conviction had been sound, based on the legal directions provided by Justice Howie, and whether Shirley Justins was entitled to an acquittal and a new trial. Eventually, they agreed that the manslaughter conviction be overturned and a new trial ordered.

Shirley Justins appealed against her conviction, but there could be no appeal against the sentence, as the facts leading to Graeme Wylie's death were not an issue.

Chief Justice Spigelman said in his judgment, 'The Crown will have the opportunity to determine whether the appellant should stand trial and, if so, whether the indictment should allege both manslaughter and aiding and abetting suicide. The appeal should be allowed, the conviction for manslaughter should be quashed and a new trial ordered'.

The decision to proceed with another trial was left up to the Director of Public Prosecutions, but eventually the Crown decided to accept a plea of assisted suicide, and as Shirley Justins had already served the sentence, she walked free.

20
An Impatient Heir: The Weightman Murders

'The darkest hour in any man's life is when he sits down to plan how to get money without earning it.'
~ *Horace Greeley*

At about 9.55 am, on Sunday, 9 January 2000, a park ranger for the Royal National Park was conducting his usual patrol of the bushland adjacent to Heathcote Road, Heathcote, when he noticed a damaged section of the mesh fence in Pipeline Road, an access road into the National Park. Thinking it odd, he decided to check it out, and on further examination of the fence, he saw a green Mitsubishi Magna sedan, registration AGO 40R, hard up against a tree, about nineteen metres down the embankment. He scrambled down towards it, and to his horror, he found two people in the front cabin of the vehicle. One was male, in the driving seat, and the other was female, in the passenger seat. Both were dead.

The ranger immediately contacted the police, who arrived at the scene shortly after and made a more thorough investigation of the vehicle and its occupants. The male driver, who wasn't wearing a seat belt, was wedged under the dashboard of the vehicle and the steering wheel, while the female's body was held up by her seatbelt, with her head resting against the front passenger window. The key was in the ignition, in the 'on' position and the engine was cold. Photographs of the vehicle with its deceased occupants in situ were taken.

Damage was confined to the front of the vehicle, but curiously, there were no skid marks on the road approaching the embankment and no damage to the guard rail before the entrance to the park.

After examining the contents of the car, police were able to identify the victims as Pamela Weightman, age fifty, and her husband, William Weightman, age fifty-one. Their bodies were taken to the Glebe mortuary, where they were formally identified by Alan Urwin and his wife, Margaret – Pamela Weightman's sister. They were called in to make the identification because the police were unable to locate Weightman's only adoptive child, twenty-year-old David, who lived with them in Glen Alpine, south-west Sydney. After viewing the bodies, Alan Urwin said the Weightmans looked as though they'd been in a fight rather than a car accident. 'Pam's hair was matted and Bill looked as though he'd been punched in the mouth and eye.'

The Urwins then set about tracking down David, finally finding him at a friend's house. When they broke the news to him, he just shrugged his shoulders before going back home with them. He didn't so much as enquire into the details surrounding his parents' death, which the Urwin's thought odd, and the following day, he astonished them even further by putting his parents' house on the market.

When the Urwins went round to the Weightman's house to check everything was in order, they saw Pam's jewellery, including her wedding ring, placed near a computer. Margaret, who was very close to her sister, said, 'She (Pam) wouldn't go out without her wedding ring'.

The day after the bodies were found, they were both subjected to post-mortems by Dr Allan Cala, a pathologist. The results revealed that William

Weightman had suffered a neck fracture consistent with striking the steering wheel, bruising to the lower legs and had inhaled vomitus. Dr Cala concluded that his death was due to the 'combined effects of positional asphyxia and inhalation of gastric contents'.

The examination of Pamela Weightman's body revealed bruising to her head, arms, legs and – surprisingly – her toes. She had also inhaled vomitus. In Dr Cala's report, he wrote, 'A puzzling feature is the presence of numerous bruises of varying ages on the hands and forearms. However, there is no positive evidence to indicate foul play at this time'. He concluded that the cause of death was due to the 'combined effects of blunt force head injury and aspiration of gastric contents'.

Blood samples were taken from the deceased. William Weightman's was found to contain:

- promethazine 0.03 milligrams per litre,
- pseudoephedrine 0.02 milligrams per litre,
- temazepam 0.2 milligrams per litre, and
- citalopram less than 0.1 milligrams per litre and no alcohol.

Pamela Weightman's was found to contain temazepam less than 0.1 milligrams per litre. Again, there was no alcohol.

The results were not significant from a toxicological point of view and I concluded that their deaths were not related to the medication found in the samples.

On 30 May 2000, an inquest into their deaths was held at Glebe Coroner's Court. The court was told that the vehicle containing the deceased persons had been found part way down an embankment, lodged against a tree, and that the Weightmans appeared to have been dead for some hours, as rigor mortis had set in.

The earlier evidence relied heavily on the post-mortem reports of Dr Allan Cala. At the time, the coroner found that William Weightman's death was due to the 'combined effects of positional asphyxia and inhalation of gastric contents as a result of a motor vehicle accident,' while Pamela Weightman's was caused by the 'combined effects of blunt force head injury and aspiration of gastric contents as a result of a motor vehicle accident'.

Other than that, all that could be established at the time was that their vehicle had driven off the road, possibly as a result of some medical ailment, such as an asthma attack being suffered by the driver, William Weightman.

When examined, the vehicle displayed damage to the front and rear nearside, where it appeared to have collided with some small trees, because those panels had bits of plant debris attached to them. There were no skid marks on the road or gravel, and no marks on the Armco guard rail.

However, the Urwins weren't happy with the findings, and their suspicions were further aroused after viewing the accident scene. Margaret Urwin said William had been a very careful driver with an excellent driving record and that he'd normally worn a seatbelt. Alan Urwin commented, 'I'm just a humble boilermaker, with no training of any detective work, but it looked wrong to me'.

The following day, they went to the Campbelltown police to express their concerns and suspicions that their nephew, David Weightman, had been involved in his parents' deaths. In a statement, dated 11 January, Margaret Urwin said, 'The accident all appears very strange to me, as I cannot imagine why they were on Heathcote Road, or how the accident could have possibly occurred'.

In June 2001, after several consultations, which included the homicide unit and the coroner, Strike Force Tenos was setup to re-investigate the Weightman deaths. Dr Allan Cala was asked to review the case, and discovered to his surprise that he had made an incredible error, as he had concluded that Pamela Weightman had died from massive head injuries, when, in fact, he'd been examining someone else's brain! That cast further doubt on the nature of her death, and by inference, that of her husband.

David Weightman received his inheritance over a period of time from the end of 2000 to early 2001. At the same time, rumours started to circulate from his circle of friends and various other community sources that he'd been involved in the murder of his parents.

Other rumours and innuendo suggested that Weightman had poisoned them using extracts from a poisonous plant found in Centennial Park.

The latter story had little evidence to support it, but along with all the other information coming to the notice of Campbelltown police and the persistence of the Urwins, it helped in the setting up of the strike force.

Many people were interviewed and statements obtained, and on 15 November 2002, David Weightman was formally interviewed by way of an ERISP (Electronically Recorded Interview of a Suspected Person) at Campbelltown police station. During the interview, he denied any involvement in the deaths of his parents, despite word that he'd earlier boasted to his friends that he'd got away with their murder. Four days later, his alleged accomplice, Terry Donai, was also interviewed, but he, too, denied any involvement.

Following the death of the Weightmans, over a period of nearly two years, David Weightman became more reckless, managing to spend about five hundred thousand dollars on drugs, overseas travel and motorbikes, all of which only added fuel to the fire of suspicion that the Urwins were burning.

Then, a further two years later, on 1 February, 2004, four years after the deaths of Bill and Pam Weightman, David admitted his foul deed to a shocked, but not overly surprised, Margaret and Alan Urwin. He told them that he and a friend, Terry Donai, had murdered his parents because they wouldn't let him buy a motorbike. He said, 'The motorbike was the icing on the cake'.

The Urwins promptly notified the police, who took David into custody at Campbelltown police station. Part 10A of the Crimes Act was read and explained to him by the custody officer, Detective Sergeant Robert Morley, and he was again formally interviewed by an ERISP, freely admitting his involvement in the murder of his parents. He then described how he had discussed murdering his parents for their estate and money, which would go to him as the sole heir, and told the police exactly how, when and where it was done.

He and Terry Donai had agreed the best way was to sedate David Weightman's parents and then suffocate them to death ('confixiation') with a pillow. He said he'd arrived at his parent's address on Abington Crescent, Glen Alpine, at about 8 pm on Saturday, 8 January 2000 with Terry Donai, whose reward for his help was to be the gift of a particular motorbike.

David Weightman had then prepared a cup of tea for each of his parents, to which he'd added some Serepax tablets, and after they'd dissolved, he'd given one to his mother, who had been in her bedroom upstairs, and one to his father, who had been relaxing in the lounge downstairs.

Weightman said, 'I didn't want them to feel any pain and I didn't want to be involved, because I didn't want to have nightmares or be haunted by it'.

He'd then left the house and waited outside while Donai had gone in to carry out the 'dirty work' of suffocating his parents. A female scream had told him his mother had been first, and shortly after, Donai had appeared, perspiring heavily. He'd said, 'That took a lot out of me and I need a hand with your dad'.

They'd both gone back into the house, where Weightman's father had been lying in a semi-conscious state in the lounge. Donai had grabbed a pillow and put it over the face of the semi-conscious man, telling Weightman to hold his father's legs to stop him struggling. Eventually, his body had become still.

They'd then loaded the two bodies into the green Mitsubishi Magna sedan, which had been parked in the garage of the house, and Donai had driven them to the place where they would eventually be discovered, with the dead mother in the front passenger seat and the dead father in the back seat. Weightman had followed in his mother's white Hyundai coupe. On reaching their destination, they'd pulled over and parked the vehicles, with the Magna facing a drop down the embankment.

Donai had then got out of the Magna and placed William Weightman in the driver's seat, leaving the ignition in the 'on' position. Donai and Weightman had then pushed the vehicle down the embankment.

After seeing it hurtle on its downward path, the two conspirators had climbed into the Hyundai and driven back to the crime scene. There, they'd drunk beer, smoked some cannabis and played pool. Donai had taken the incriminating pillow with him when he'd left, early the next morning, in his car.

David Weightman's confession was subject to a media suppression order and an undercover investigation was initiated. Weightman was subsequently charged and held in custody, where his case was mentioned before the courts with the order in place. That was done to ensure that the confidentiality wouldn't compromise further investigations into Donai's involvement in the murders. The order remained in place until Donai's conviction four years later.

In the meantime, the autopsy findings of William and Pamela Weightman had been re-assessed by Dr Kevin Lee of Monash University, who wrote in his summary:

> In both the case(s) of Pamela and William Weightman, there are a series of injuries which are of a pattern resembling those of a scuffle, including pinioning or moving. In each case there is not significant and incontrovertible motor vehicle accident-type damage. This is in keeping with the recognised low impact in this case. Both persons show some evidence of an asphyxia mode of death, with William Weightman having laryngeal fractures. William Weightman shows evidence of having been positioned within the car, rather than having been in a normal driving situation at the time of the incident. Neither person shows any evidence of having made any attempt to rescue themselves after this incident; this being one in which a single fatal outcome, and even more so a double fatal outcome, would appear most unlikely.

This finding was independently supported by an accident reconstruction expert, Sergeant John Kelly, who reviewed the available material gathered from the crime scene in the National Park where the Weightmans appeared to have died. In his report, dated 16 October 2003, he wrote, 'Given the minor nature of the collision, one would expect injuries to both occupants would be relatively minor if any. Although the occupants would experience a bumpy ride down the embankment, the final impact is equivalent to most minor collisions which occur across Sydney each day generally without injury. Therefore, given this, it is unlikely that the collision led, or contributed, to their deaths'.

Essentially, those findings supported the admissions of David Weightman as well as the suspicions of the Urwins.

While David Weightman was in custody, the police continued to concentrate their inquiries into the movements of Terry Donai, who had since moved to the town of Cooma, NSW. There, he formed a series of relationships with different women, one of whom was financially independent. She eventually tired of the one-sided relationship and required police assistance to get him to move on. Undeterred, Donai formed another relationship with a much younger woman, and together, along with Donai's young son from a previous relationship, they moved into rented premises in Cooma, where he did casual work while still collecting social security benefits. All the time, he was totally unaware of the covert evidence gathering team that had been assembled in conjunction with Cooma and Queanbeyan detectives. In September 2005, they set up an intercept for Donai's mobile and landline calls, together with physical surveillance to determine his movements, associates and habits.

David Weightman's trial was approaching rapidly, and the police intercepted a number of calls between Terry Donai and others relating to it. It became apparent from listening to those conversations that Donai had something to hide. Fortunately, the media suppression order was in place and his access to sensitive information was limited.

On the day of his murder trial, David Weightman appeared before Justice Hidden and surprisingly entered a plea of guilty. He was then remanded in custody, at which time, the judge deferred sentencing until just before Christmas, 2005. That provided the police with a further opportunity to gather more information through their covert operations unit.

On 23 December 2005, David Weightman appeared once more before Justice Hidden and was sentenced to forty years gaol for the murder of his parents. However, Justice Hidden ruled that because Weightman had pleaded guilty, shown co-operation and assisted the police, he was going to reduce the sentence. He then ruled that, 'The offender is sentenced for the murder of his father to imprisonment for twenty-five years, with a non-parole period of nineteen years, to date from 2 February, 2004. For the murder of his mother, he is sentenced to imprisonment for twenty-five years, with a non-parole period of nineteen years, to date from 2 February 2007. He will be eligible for release on parole on 1 February 2026'. Both sentences were to run concurrently, so essentially, Weightman was sentenced to twenty-five years for the murders of both his adoptive parents, with a non-parole period of nineteen years.

During the investigation, Donai met with a number of covert operatives, who gained some disturbing insights into the man. On one occasion he was recorded as telling one operative that if Weightman were dead, they'd have nothing on him.

On 16 June 2006, Donai met up with a further two operatives in Sydney. During their meeting, he detailed his knowledge and involvement in the murders of the Weightmans, explaining how they'd been killed and that David had assisted him in transferring and disposing of their bodies in Bill's Magna, which had been pushed down an embankment in order to give the impression that a motor vehicle accident had caused the couple's deaths. He was subsequently arrested and taken to Maroubra police station, where, on legal advice, he refused to be interviewed. However, given his previous comments to an operative about Weightman and the fact that he had a relative working with the corrective services department, David Weightman was placed into protective custody.

The following day, Donai appeared before Parramatta Local Court, where he was refused bail and remanded in custody. He was then transferred to the Metropolitan Remand and Reception Centre, commonly known as the MRRC, which forms part of the Silverwater correctional complex, located at Holker Street, Silverwater, Sydney, NSW. During that time, police continued to monitor Donai's telephone calls, which were to prove useful in determining his financial position and motivation for committing the crimes.

Terry Donai's trial got underway on a warm Monday morning on 17 September 2007 before Her Honour, Justice Elizabeth Fullerton, at the Supreme Court, Taylor Square, Darlinghurst.

The Supreme Court sits in a fine old heritage-listed sandstone building, which has witnessed many a great court battle. Donai's trial was to be no exception.

After the usual opening addresses to the jury and some *voir dires* to establish witness reliability, the trial began with family and friends of the Weightmans giving evidence, most of which went largely unchallenged. However, the vital evidence was to be drawn from David Weightman and the admissions given by Terry Donai to undercover police.

Weightman was subjected to intense questioning and gave evidence that was consistent with his ERISP interviews. I also gave evidence which supported Weightman's version and Donai's admissions, but indicated that the levels of drugs found in the Weightman's bodies had had no bearing on their deaths. In my view, the levels detected had been too low to have had any appreciable level of sedation, which rather made nonsense out of David Weightman's earlier comment, when he'd said, 'I didn't want them to feel any pain and I didn't want to be involved, because I didn't want to have nightmares or be haunted by it'. Furthermore, the low levels I found showed that his mother would have appeared to have suffered the most.

During the trial, various documents were presented in evidence, including telephone and banking records. Evidence showing that Donai had used several young women to live off their earnings was also submitted. He'd been a total 'grub' before moving on to murder. However, a significant factor raised during the trial was the use of the covert investigation techniques. While the media suppression order was still in place, various media sought to have it lifted so they could report on the matter, but the Commissioner of Police, Mr Andrew Scipione, lodged an appeal to have an interim order to have the suppression order remain in place. The matter went before the Court of Criminal Appeal, which agreed it should remain. That decision was appealed, but only overturned by the High Court, ruling in favour of the media, after Donai's trial.

On Thursday, 11 October 2007, after various closing addresses from the prosecution and defence, the jury retired to consider their verdict. They returned the following Monday, 15 October, with verdicts of guilty for the murders of both Pamela and William Weightman. However, they were not requested to find verdicts on the alternative charges of being an accessory after the fact to murder.

Sentencing was fixed for 23 May 2008 and Donai was remanded in custody to await his fate. When the day came round, he appeared before the same judge in courtroom number two of the King Street Supreme Court, in Sydney, NSW. It's quite a small court, but it's been the setting for many human dramas that have played out over the years, from serial rapes to murder.

Margaret and Alan Urwin sat a short distance from Donai, who was seated in the dock. They were keen to see his face when, hopefully, a lengthy gaol sentence would be handed down.

Justice Fullerton delivered her judgment on the sentence, saying during her submission that Mrs Urwin had described her sister and husband Bill as irreplaceable family members and valued citizens of the community who had both been stolen from her. 'I am satisfied that this has occasioned her the deepest grief and has been productive of deep and enduring trauma which has shattered her family and eventually led to a breakdown in her marriage.' She continued, 'The extent of this offender's blatant disregard for common decency and his patent disrespect for the integrity and sanctity of human life is breathtaking. The real question, it seems to me, is whether or not there is any basis for this offender being described as anything other than a killer under contract. However, I am satisfied that this offender proposed the method of killing and the means of its successful execution in the expectation that he would receive a reward and, as the evidence reveals, he took steps over many months after their deaths to extract what he regarded as being due to him'.

In determining the sentence, Her Honour said, 'The community at large is, however, entitled to look to this court for the imposition of a sentence which meets its legitimate desire for retribution when two of its community members have been senselessly and heartlessly killed as they approached the end of a productive and honest working life. It hardly needs emphasis from me that the community is entitled to have the sentence imposed on this offender to produce the effect, if only in the abstract, of deterring others from taking life for the promise of financial reward. I sentence Terry Mark Donai to concurrent sentences of imprisonment for life, each to date from 16 June, 2006'.

Donai stood ashen faced in the dock, in contrast to the Urwins, whose reaction was one of relief, exhilaration and at last, a sense of closure. It appeared to be a done deal and justice had finally been served.

Unfortunately, that was not to be.

Incredibly, the matter went to a court of appeal and the first conviction was quashed (overturned) because the evidence provided by a secretly recorded confession to an undercover police officer appeared to cause a miscarriage of justice! Donai was subsequently granted a re-trial. The Urwins were aghast, saying outside the court, 'We thought he didn't have a chance in hell of getting a new trial'.

It was going to be another six long years before justice was truly administered. When the day of reckoning finally arrived, the matter appeared before Justice Peter Hidden, and the crown prosecutors, Ms Margaret Cunneen, Senior Counsel, and Ms Justine Hopper, had a difficult job ahead of them as the Court of Criminal Appeal had thrown out fifty per cent of the evidence, meaning they had to conduct the second trial with both hands tied behind their backs. But these were no ordinary women, and they put together a convincing brief of evidence.

David Weightman gave evidence at both trials, telling the court that Terry Donai had offered to kill his adopted parents for seventeen thousand dollars, which he'd intended to use to purchase a motorcycle. He admitted that he'd drugged his parents in the hope they wouldn't suffer and that he'd assisted Donai in the suffocation of his father.

Terry Donai was once again found guilty.

In her sentencing submissions, Deputy Senior Crown Prosecutor, Margaret Cunneen, Senior Counsel, said Donai should receive the maximum sentence because he'd been motivated only by greed and had shown no remorse.

In sentencing Donai, Justice Peter Hidden said, 'In the sanctity of their home, Mr and Mrs Weightman were killed in a brutal manner. I am particularly conscious of the agony she and the family must have suffered waiting so long for this offender to come to justice'. He then sentenced Donai to a maximum of forty years, with a non-parole period of thirty years for each offence.

Outside the court, Alan and Margaret Urwin said that Donai should have received two life sentences, as handed down by Justice Elizabeth Fullerton earlier in 2007. Alan Urwin said, 'The sentence was not appropriate, but as I say, this should have been handed down over ten years ago. I'm asking the Premier for a full and independent investigation into this to determine why NSW Police refused to investigate an obvious double murder, which they left to the family to get evidence to get two murderers brought to justice in NSW. For four years, we had to do the job for NSW Police. For four years, they were telling us that this was a motor vehicle accident, that we were being paranoid, and to get on with our life. There was no evidence to suggest this was a motor vehicle accident – all the evidence pointed to a murder'.

A visibly shaken, Margaret Urwin added, 'Nothing is going to bring Pam and Bill back, so you don't move on, you live with it'.

A victim's advocate, Mr Howard Brown, said, 'This was a crime committed purely for profit, for no other reason, and if that doesn't fall into the worst case category and deserve a life sentence for both murders, I don't know what we expect of our judicial system anymore'.

Terry Donai will be eligible for parole on 15th June 2039.

The case took its toll on the Urwin family, as Alan and Margaret Urwin divorced and went their separate ways. As for getting an independent inquiry into the handling of case that the Urwins demanded, the New South Wales Premier ruled it out, saying that the matter had been finalised as the two offenders were now behind bars.

However, something worthwhile did come out of the case in that there have since been significant changes made to call out procedures for the crash investigation unit and the management of crime scenes associated with suspicious motor vehicle accidents.

21 Mystery Cliff Top Fall: The Sarah Rawson Case

'When ill luck begins,
it does not come in sprinkles, but in showers.'
~ ***Mark Twain***

Hargraves Lookout, a small, uneven rocky outcrop that provides magnificent views over the rural Megalong Valley is located at the southern end of Shipley Plateau, Blackheath, in the Blue Mountains of New South Wales. It was named in honour of William Henry Hargraves (1839-1925), the Deputy Registrar in Equity, who was once known as the father of Blackheath. However, in spite of its rugged beauty, it used to be a very dangerous place for the unwary, as there was no barrier or fence between the ledge and a sheer cliff drop of several hundred metres.

It's against this background that this story unfolds.

At about 11.30 am on 11 March, 2006, twenty-three-year-old Shawn Mullen picked up Sarah Rawson, his new girlfriend of three weeks, from her home in Cambridge Park, Penrith, Sydney. She was an attractive young lady, two years Mullen's senior. They were just like any other regular dating couple, except for the fact that Sarah was wheelchair bound, having been involved in a horrific head-on car crash four months earlier, outside Ballina, NSW, which had resulted in thirty-five broken bones, including both arms and legs. Since then she'd relied on a wheelchair for mobility of more than a few metres, and only used crutches when absolutely necessary, as that method of movement proved to be more painful for her. But she wasn't one to brood about the unfairness of the world, and was determined to get on with her life, even booking a South Pacific cruise with her mother, who'd been helping her recover. Sarah was an easy going social educator, who worked with disabled and mentally ill people. She was very popular and enjoyed life, often being described as vibrant and beautiful.

It was their fourth date, and they spent a few hours sightseeing in Katoomba before deciding to have an early evening picnic at Hargraves Lookout. After buying a bottle of Omni Pink sparkling wine, a packet of crackers, some cheese and a few strawberries, Shawn placed Sarah into the passenger seat of his grey Holden Rodeo utility before loading her wheelchair into the back, along with the food and drink.

It was late afternoon when they arrived at their destination, and the area was deserted. An early evening mist was creeping up the Megalong Valley, the silence only being broken by the occasional sound from the bush birdlife. A peaceful, idyllic location. Shawn unloaded the vehicle and placed a picnic rug a few metres from the edge of the cliff. After helping Sarah onto the rug, the 'bubbly' was popped and the pair settled down to dine on the wine, cheese and crackers while enjoying the spectacular views over the valley below.

Around 5.45 pm, Sarah told Shawn that she needed to make 'a call of nature' and asked him to look away, which he did. While his head was turned the other way, he heard a little scream, and when he turned back, Sarah was gone, having fallen seventy metres to her death over the cliff edge.

Mullen immediately rang 000, outlining to the operator what had happened.

A police rescue team arrived, along with detectives and crime scene officers who examined the area, taking photographs of the scene, Shawn Mullen's grey Holden Rodeo utility and Sarah's body in its final resting place.

The rescue officers and forensic experts then abseiled down the cliff to examine Sarah's body, which was only winched up from the base of the cliff the following day because bad weather and poor visibility hampered its retrieval at the time. After gathering as much evidence as they could and taking a statement from Shawn Mullen, police went to inform Sarah's mother. Unfortunately, the timing couldn't have been worse. Margaret Rawson had arranged a party in her daughter's honour, and she and about fifty guests were waiting for Sarah to arrive.

What should have been a celebration of her life turned into a night of grief-stricken anguish.

After formal identification, Sarah's body was taken to the Department of Forensic Medicine, Westmead Hospital for a post-mortem, which was carried out by Dr Peter SJ Ellis.

He concluded that, 'Death was due to the effect of multiple injuries (described previously in the report) of which the most serious were severe head injury and damage to the neck and chest. These are consistent with the alleged fall from a cliff. While blood and urine alcohol were elevated, there was nothing in the autopsy to suggest (or exclude) any altercation prior to the fall'.

It was quite a conservative report.

Sarah's funeral took place on a cold, drizzly Monday on 20 March 2006. The service was attended by family and friends, and her ashes were later scattered in Ballina, a town she loved and where she'd been planning to open a shop when she recovered from her injuries. Shawn Mullen didn't attend the funeral or see Sarah's family despite having previously said he was devastated by her death.

Carl Milovanovich, the deputy state coroner, conducted an inquest on 11 May 2009. At the centre of the enquiry was how mobile Sarah had been on the day of her death.

Shawn Mullen was the last person to have seen Sarah alive and he reiterated what he'd previously told police about his and Sarah's date up to the point when she disappeared over the cliff. He said how, despite her disability, he'd helped her over the barrier at the lookout, three metres from the edge of the cliff, before returning to his utility at close on 5.45 pm to collect her wheelchair, also claiming that she'd been keen to look around after being carried to the cliff edge. He told the inquest that he and Sarah had been intimate, after which she'd asked him to turn away while she urinated, even though there had been a toilet only a short distance away. He admitted he'd glanced back and seen that she'd been trying to pull up her jeans, but hadn't seen her fall. He'd then made the 000 call.

The coroner heard evidence that Sarah Rawson's worried friends had tried to warn her off Shawn Mullen a week before her death, calling him a 'psycho'. That seemed to be supported by Mullen's friends who said he was unusual, and also described him as obsessive and weird.

Detective Senior Constable John Fasano provided evidence that a former girlfriend of Shawn Mullen had dumped him because of his violent mood swings, saying, 'She stated that his depressive mood swings and raging temper stopped their relationship'.

The coroner was also told that Shawn Mullen had twice been admitted to Paella psychiatric ward for treatment and that he had a history of mental illness, going back to 2001.

Detective Senior Constable Fasano also said he thought it strange that Sarah Rawson hadn't attempted to use the toilet that was about twenty-five metres away. In his view, he felt, 'It would be odd for a female to go to the toilet on the edge of a cliff without any toilet paper and in full view of any person who could have driven down the road at any time'. However, he admitted he'd been unable to determine whether the toilet had been operational or open on the day Sarah had died.

Another police witness, Detective Senior Constable Jason Howe told the court, 'He (Mullen) heard a little scream, turned around and she was gone. In relation to the 000 call, he said that Mullen had asked if he would be charged with manslaughter before saying that he thought he'd be going to jail and that Sarah's body was in four pieces. Then Mullen had said he couldn't see her, and that he'd have to notify her parents, who would think it was his fault'.

The detective then put before the inquest three possible scenarios:

'Firstly, Rawson fell from the cliff in the manner that Mullen described. Secondly, and to my mind, equally likely, Mullen pushed her over the cliff. Finally, Rawson was being assisted back from the cliff edge by Mullen and he accidentally dropped her, causing her to fall over the edge. That may have caused Mullen to construct a story to cover his perceived recklessness or negligence.'

A number of other witnesses came forward and gave evidence in relation to the case, including myself. I was at the inquest to interpret the levels of drugs and alcohol detected in Sarah Rawson's blood sample, and so determine how much she would have been affected at the time of the tragedy. Shawn Mullen had previously said that Sarah Rawson had consumed two schooners of Tooheys New full-strength beer between 1 pm and 3 pm and more than half of the 750 ml bottle of Omni Pink (11.5 per cent alcohol) sparkling wine just prior to her death. Sarah had been used to drinking alcohol and had been taking the drug sertraline for four weeks. The analyst's reports, carried out by the Division of Analytical Laboratories, Lidcombe, New South Wales, showed the following levels of the drug and alcohol in the blood sample taken at post mortem: sertraline 0.2 milligram per litre and alcohol 0.150 grams per decilitre (100 millilitres) of blood. Her urine sample was found to have present alcohol 0.208 grams per decilitre (100 millilitres) of urine. I calculated Sarah's likely blood alcohol level at the time of her death to have been 0.150 grams per decilitre, and found to my surprise that the drinking history the inquest had been provided with to be quite accurate. (Quite often, they're either understated or overstated, depending upon the circumstances!)

I told the inquest that level of sertraline or Zoloft was not an issue, as Sarah had been taking the drug for about four weeks to treat anxiety and depression and it was within the therapeutic level needed for treatment of that condition. However, the level of alcohol in her blood would have affected her faculties, and given her proximity to the cliff edge, impaired her ability to react effectively in an emergency situation. Essentially, she would have been under the influence of alcohol and in a very vulnerable situation which could have led to the fatal outcome.

After some consideration, Carl Milovanovich found that Sarah Rawson had died from multiple injuries following an accidental fall from a cliff edge at Hargraves Lookout, near Blackheath, on 11 March 2006. He commented, 'Having examined all the evidence, it is the view of this court that Sarah's death was a tragic accident'. He also recommended that Blue Mountains City Council examine the site where Sarah had fallen to her death and consider more fencing and better signage because of its proximity to a car park. He said, 'My concern is that this rock ledge is adjacent to a car park and young children could easily run out of vehicles or wander into this area and not be aware of the potential danger. Similarly, adults may not be aware of the sudden cliff drop and the uneven surface'.

Since the coroner recommendation to Blue Mountains City Council, only a token barrier fence has been erected adjacent to the car park, and a sign on a pole, depicting a stick figure in danger, has been placed at the tragic site in lieu of a safety fence.

While it is a beautiful scene over the Megalong Valley, I personally believe a barrier fence should be installed to protect the foolhardy and to respect the death of a beautiful young Australian woman. Perhaps a plaque should be erected in her memory – which may also provide a warning to other visitors to the site.

22 Sex, Drugs and a Body in the Bush

'Man is the cruellest animal.'
~ Friedrich Nietzsche

Pia Kate Navida was an attractive Filipino teenager who migrated to Australia from the Philippines in the early 1980s as a very young bride of an Australian national. Treasured by her family, she was a young woman full of hope and promise. Physically, she was a real stunner, with a shapely body, beautiful golden skin, almond-shaped eyes and lovely dark hair. But underneath all that outward beauty lurked a fiery temper. Eventually, her somewhat laid-back husband couldn't take her outbursts anymore and they divorced, leaving Pia in a terrible financial situation. To make ends meet, she resorted to prostitution and adopted a nomadic lifestyle, which brought her into contact with a number of undesirables and led her to embrace the drug scene, in particular, the stimulant methylamphetamine (also known as speed).

Her favourite haunts were in the area around Sydney Central railway station, where she solicited for sex in bars, as well as at Greasey's Cafe in Elizabeth Street, a short walk away. She had several boyfriends, but treated them more as a convenience to herself than as partners in a satisfying mutual relationship. Rather than pleasing her lovers, it was more a case of them pleasing her. Perhaps her work as a prostitute made her feel it was her turn for some enjoyment.

At 1 pm, on Friday, 31 January 1992, she was at the Central Station bar, having drinks with friends, when she met up with a potential customer who offered her a lift. She accepted, and that was the last time she was seen alive.

The following day, around twelve o'clock, some bushwalkers were trekking by Bundeena, a quaint village surrounded by the Royal National Park on the outskirts of southern Sydney, about twenty-nine kilometres from Sydney central business district, when they came across some clothing scattered across the bush track. An orange coloured face washer hung on a branch nearby.

Puzzling over where the clothing might have come from, the walkers soon stumbled upon the battered naked body of Pia Navida. It was on a service track known as Marley's Beach Trail. She was lying on her back and it looked like she'd been bludgeoned to death. A large fourteen-kilogram bloodstained sandstone rock, the probable murder weapon, lay nearby. The police were promptly called, the area sealed off and the witnesses interviewed. It was determined she'd been raped and then bludgeoned to death with the large sandstone rock, which had crushed her face, making her barely recognisable. Her body had then been dragged a short distance and dumped.

After her body had been taken to the Glebe morgue in Sydney, the police investigation began in earnest. Strike Force Ever, comprising detectives from the state crime command's unsolved homicide team, was established to investigate the circumstances surrounding her death.

Investigating police were certain that more than one culprit had been involved, and a number of suspects, including Wayne Taylor – a man with whom she'd had a somewhat volatile, and at times violent, relationship – were investigated and cleared. Sadly, the investigation then appeared to have reached a dead end.

A number of samples were taken from Pia's body at the post-mortem for toxicological examination.

Her blood sample was found to have present:

- methylamphetamine 1.0 milligram per litre, and
- pseudoephedrine 0.15 milligram per litre.

A liver sample was found to contain:

- 0.2 milligram per kilogram of methylamphetamine.

Her stomach sample was found to have present:

- 0.23 milligram per litre of methylamphetamine, and
- 0.07 milligram of pseudoephedrine.

Her urine sample was found to contain:

- 13 milligrams per litre of methylamphetamine,
- pseudoephedrine 7.3 milligrams per litre, and
- cannabinoids (cannabis products).

This toxicology profile provided a number of pieces of evidence that I later provided to the Supreme Court at Taylor Square, Darlinghurst.

Firstly, her blood level for methylamphetamine (meth) showed she'd clearly been a seasoned meth user. The therapeutic range (the 'feel good' level) for this drug is 0.01 to 0.05 milligram per litre. Pia's blood level was well outside this range. The pseudoephedrine could have come from a number of sources, an impurity in the original methylamphetamine source or from a flu medication. However, methylamphetamine is readily synthesised from pseudoephedrine.

Secondly, the presence of the drug in her stomach contents indicated that she had taken the drug orally, and because some of it was still there (it hadn't all been absorbed into her blood stream), it indicated recent usage. Methylamphetamine can be taken orally (by mouth), intra nasally (snorting the powder), injected or by smoking. Users may become dependent upon the drug and use it with increasing frequency and in larger doses to get the same desired effect.

Additional forensic samples, including swabs and fingernail clippings were also taken from Pia's body at the post-mortem. Those specimens were stored in a refrigerator and later proved to be very useful for further future (cold case) investigations into the murder.

In 1994, an inquest into Pia's death was held, returning an open finding as to who took her life under such brutal circumstances. And there the matter lay until much needed advances in DNA technology took place.

But fortunately, science never rests, and twelve years later, an identifiable DNA profile was extracted from the semen swabs taken from both the interior and exterior of Pia Navida's body. The profiles were uploaded into the now established national DNA database, which had begun to yield some very worthwhile results for a number of cold cases, and matches were made with a man known as Steven Isaac Matthews and another two males. Unfortunately, the evidence didn't appear to be sufficient to convict the suspects, but with further testing, in 2011, it was found that semen swab samples taken from Pia's body were consistent with the DNA profiles of two males, Rodney James Paterson and Steven Isaac Matthews.

It appeared that both Steven Matthews and Rodney Paterson had had sex with Pia Navida prior to her death, but police still had to ascertain who had done the final foul deed. The crime scene had seemed to indicate more than one participant was involved, so the police swung into action and arrested both men.

Rodney Paterson, who was arrested in Bathurst, first appeared at Bathurst Local Court. He didn't apply for bail, which had been formally refused anyway, and reappeared at the Central Local Court in Sydney. In the meantime, police successfully sought the extradition of Steven Matthews, who was arrested near Melbourne, in Melbourne Magistrate's Court. He was then transported across the border to Albury, where he was formally charged at Albury Local Court with murder and sexual assault. As expected, bail was refused. The matter then went before the Supreme Court in court seven, Taylor Square, Darlinghurst before Justice Geoffrey Bellew, on 3 February 2014.

That was just over twenty-two years after Pia Navida's violent sexual assault and murder.

Matthews pleaded guilty to both rape and murder. He even said that he'd taken a girlfriend for picnics to Bundeena, where Pia Navida's body had been found, and told her he'd killed a person in the bush area before showing her how he'd carried it out. He also told the court that he, too, had been a victim of a major assault, in 2005, which had left him with a serious brain injury and little memory of his earlier life.

Paterson maintained his innocence regarding both charges. He initially denied knowing Pia Navida, although he did admit he might have met her at the bar she used to frequent near the Central railway station. However, he later changed his story, stating that he had, in fact, had consensual sex with her before her death.

The Crown pointed out that Paterson's DNA had been found under Pia Navida's finger nails, in her anus and on her right breast, which suggested a struggle, but John Stratton, Senior Counsel for the defence, said that even if the DNA evidence proved that Paterson had had anal sex with Pia, it didn't prove that he'd had any role in her rape or murder, or that he'd been at the scene when the crime had occurred.

Stratton asked Justice Bellew to direct the jury to enter verdicts of not guilty on both charges on the grounds that 'even at its highest, the evidence was incapable of convincing the jury that my client was guilty'.

On consideration, Justice Bellew upheld the application, and instructed the jury to acquit Rodney Paterson on both charges, saying, 'Although the evidence is capable of placing the accused at the scene at the relevant time, it says nothing at all about his participation in the act which caused the deceased's death. Presence at the scene does not sustain an inference in the killing of the deceased'.

Furthermore, drawing from the forensic pathologist, Dr Johan Duflou, who carried out the post-mortem on Pia Navida's body, Justice Bellew also found that there was a lack of evidence to support the Crown's case that there had been a struggle between the two, prior to her death. He commented, 'I am not satisfied that the existence of a broken rib, and the presence of the accused's DNA on the deceased fingernails, in combination with the other matters relied upon by the Crown, sustain an interference that a struggle took place. There were no injuries suggestive of forced intercourse, nor any external injury, such as bruising'.

As for the lies Paterson had told the police, Justice Bellew said, 'While it may be that he answered questions put by the police because he did not wish to connect himself with the events surrounding the deceased's death that does not, without more, lead to the conclusion that his motivation for making such statements was realisation of guilt of either of the offences with which he has been charged. Indeed, there were statements made by the accused, both in the course of his second interview with the police and the two conversations with his partner, which were at odds with such a realisation'.

Following His Honour's direction, the jury acquitted Paterson, who walked from the court a free man.

In the meantime, Steven Isaac Matthews was in custody awaiting his sentencing, which came on 22 May, 2014, when Justice Geoffrey Bellew handed down a term of imprisonment of twenty-one years and six months, given the 'barbaric' and 'horrendous' nature of his crime. He was given a non-parole period of sixteen years and three months which, with time in custody, makes him eligible for parole in November 2027.

23

Anguish in Armidale: Kids and Custody

'When it comes to determining child custody, [however], sexism is the rule.'
~ Phyllis Schlafly

Armidale is a country town located in the Northern Tablelands of New South Wales, Australia. It's a charming place to visit and live, with four distinct seasons: a warm summer, colours of red, yellow and amber during the autumn, a crisp and often white winter, and a very enjoyable sparkling spring, with a riot of colour from the many flower gardens. It's also a place of world-class academia, with the University of New England offering state-of-the-art technology and educational diversity.

It was in this near idyllic setting that David Goebel McGregor, a sixty-two-year-old divorcee struck up a friendship with a much younger woman, thirty-nine-year-old Vivian Acheson. Vivian had come to Australia from England on a visitor's visa and was backpacking around the countryside when they met. David had placed an advertisement in a Sydney newspaper for help on a property he was leasing, north-west of Glen Innes, and Vivian applied and was taken on. Vivian had never been to the Australian Outback and quickly grew to love both it and David. In spite of their age difference, they started sleeping together after a week and formed a close relationship, initially moving into a fairly humble abode. Shortly afterwards, their first child, Cameron, was born. Planning to have further offspring, they took the opportunity to buy a small cottage on seven acres of land in Torrington. It was a vast improvement on their earlier residence, which had originally been without electricity and hot running water. After three months or so, Vivian suggested that since they were in a permanent relationship, she should apply for Australian visa residency, which could eventually lead to Australian citizenship. David thought that was a good idea, so she applied to the immigration department and provided the necessary details. She was granted temporary residency, and eventually, permanent residency. Things appeared to be looking up. However, Vivian had a roving eye and unbeknown to David, she'd begun an affair after their second son, Ryan, had been born.

On New Year's Day, 2001, David McGregor received a phone call that was to change his life. It was from a friend's wife, Carol Ellis.

'Hi, David, just rang to wish you a happy new year.'

David returned the greeting.

The true reason for her call then became evident. She'd kicked her husband, Doug Ellis, out of the house two weeks earlier after finding he'd been cheating on her.

'Sorry to hear that, Carol,' David replied. 'I didn't know you were having problems.'

But the worst news was yet to come.

'I'm sorry to tell you on New Year's Day, David, but he's been having an affair with Vivian for the last three months.'

Carol then said that she thought Doug had been in David and Vivian's Torrington house with their four-month-old baby boy, Ryan, as he'd rung from that address the day after Christmas Day.

David then asked Vivian about what Carol had told him. She denied there was any truth in it and said that Carol was making it up.

David then asked, 'Why would she? There's no reason for her to fabricate a story like that'. He reached for the phone and dialled, but set it down again when Vivian said, 'I don't know. Okay, it's true, so what?'

Understandably, David was hurt and felt betrayed. 'I can't live with something like that.'

Vivian just shrugged and said, 'Well, I'm going now to see Doug. I'm leaving'.

After a heated discussion, bordering on a row, Vivian left with their youngest son, Ryan, as he hadn't been weaned, leaving their other three-year-old son, Cameron, with David. As she was leaving, her parting comment was, 'I'll get the police onto you and I'm going to apply for full custody of the children'.

The following Monday, David McGregor received a summons to appear in court at Glen Innes. Vivian Acheson had applied for full custody of their children. That was followed up by an affidavit, which was presented to him at the court. Given its unexpected detrimental contents, he'd no time to prepare for a defence and had to search around to find a legal representative to act on his behalf.

The two solicitors from both sides conferred, discussing the pros and cons and the difficulty of the situation, and they asked Vivian, 'Why do you want to go for full custody? Why don't you be reasonable and let David have access to the children?'

After further discussion she relented, but not without bitterness, and an interim agreement was put into place until the next court hearing.

She told David, 'You can't win, I'm going to beat you, you know,' to which he replied, 'There's no winner or loser here, there's only losing for the children'.

David McGregor eventually moved his possessions out of his and Vivian's Torrington home into a renovated unit in Guyra. It was in a two-storey weatherboard building which had been subdivided into five self-contained flats. After several acrimonious exchanges, including the issue of an AVO, after an indiscrete comment to Vivian, where he commented, 'Now, I understand why some Australian husbands in my situation take their own lives and their wives,' the child custody issues were beginning to take their toll, and he became deeply depressed. He was advised to visit a doctor, who prescribed a hundred milligrams of Zoloft (sertraline) to treat his depression and cope with his situation. Unfortunately, he stopped taking the medication two weeks before what turned out to be the fateful afternoon in both his, Vivian's and their two children's lives.

It was a quiet Sunday afternoon on 8 December 2002. The custody battle had been going on for some time. It had been a very difficult arrangement with little or no leeway in negotiations, and the situation had become even more difficult since Vivian had taken up with Doug, her new lover, after the birth of their second child. On that Sunday afternoon, Vivian arrived at David's flat with a friend, Jeffrey Orchard, and young son, Ryan, to pick up their other son, Cameron. David was there with his business partners and friends, Mike and Kerrie-Anne Hunt, with whom he ran a Mr Whippy ice cream franchise in Armidale. After putting the kettle on to make a cup of coffee, David asked everyone, including a fellow flatmate, to leave while he and Vivian had a discussion about the on-going problem of access. The group headed off to the Guyra Tavern for a drink, leaving David and Vivian to sort out their differences. Meanwhile, the two boys were left to play in the adjacent hall and an empty flat next door. After some discussion, Vivian turned to David and said, 'If you think I came down here to pick up the boys to do you a favour, you can, but don't think I did you any favour'.

'What do you mean?' David asked.

'I'm taking the boys down to Doug's place, in Parkes, from here,' she replied. 'If it's any interest to you, because you've been whingeing about it for so long, if you must know, Ryan will be sleeping in the bed with Doug and me, and if Cameron wants to sleep in with us, he can too.'

As she drank her cup of coffee, she said, 'I told you, you can't [get access], and that I'm going to beat you.'

David McGregor had heard enough and walked out of the room, passing the two boys, who had found a toilet roll and were dragging the paper everywhere. He went over to his gun cabinet, which contained two vintage shotguns and two 22-calibre rifles, undid the padlock and took out a 22-calibre rifle. He then snapped a magazine containing ten bullets into the weapon and returned to the lounge, with the boys still playing in the adjoining room, and closed the door.

In the meantime, Vivian had gone out into the kitchen to wash her cup. Due to a creaky floorboard she heard David walk into the lounge and said, 'By the way, when I win the court case in June, Doug and I will be taking the boys to England, and you will never see them again'.

She turned with a smile that turned into a smirk.

David took one step forward and pulled the trigger of the rifle. The shot entered her head. It was instantly fatal. Vivian fell backwards, striking her head on the floor. A smell of cordite lingered in the air from the rifle discharge.

The final solution.

After a brief pause, David rang the Guyra Tavern to tell his friends that he and Vivian were still discussing custody of the children. He then collected the boys and took them down to Vivian's car, which was parked outside the back stairs of the building. He expected to find the keys in the ignition, but the car was locked. Leaving the boys near the car he said, 'Cameron, you watch Ryan for a moment'. He rushed back upstairs and, after a quick search, he found the car keys in Vivian's hand. He plucked them from her lifeless body and returned to the vehicle, bundling the boys into the back seat.

It was about 6 pm when he started the motor and headed off to Sydney. He drove out of the yard, along Bradley Street and over a railway crossing onto the New England Highway. From there, he made his way to Black Mountain, where he stopped at the Black Mountain Service Station and rang the Guyra Tavern from the public telephone. When a barmaid answered, he asked if she could page Kerrie-Anne.

A few moments later, she came to the telephone.

'Hi, David, how's things?' she asked.

'Fine,' he replied. 'You guys are welcome to take the car up to Glen Innes tonight and Mike can drive down and open up the store tomorrow.'

After the usual farewells, he got back into the vehicle, where his sons were dozing.

In the meantime, his friends decided to call it a night and return to the unit, where they found Vivian's body in the kitchen with a single gunshot wound to the back of her head. Armidale police were notified, and when they arrived at the scene, they conducted their normal investigation in such a situation and seized a number of firearms before having Vivian's body transported to the morgue.

It was going to be a long night for David and his boys. As the fuel tank was almost full, no further purchase was necessary, and they continued their journey on to Muswellbrook, a trip of about three and a half to four hours. By the time they arrived, it was quite dark and the moon was only a thin crescent in the sky. They pulled into the Muswellbrook Service Station, where David refuelled and bought little packets of Smarties along with little cartons of fruit juice for the boys. The next stop was at the Singleton Service Station, where he bought sausage rolls for a late evening meal, and then it was on to Ryde, Sydney, where his daughter lived.

At around 2 am, they pulled into the driveway of her home. His surprised daughter met him at the door. 'Dad, what's going on?'

'Hi, dear, I've brought the children down. I just want to stay the night. There's been a bit of trouble. I'm exhausted.'

His daughter took them to a spare bedroom, where there was large bed for the three of them to spend the night. After putting the sleepy boys to bed, David said to his daughter, 'In the morning, we'll talk about it. I just wanna have some sleep now'.

'Okay, Dad, tomorrow. Good night.'

David McGregor had a very restless night, but the boys slept soundly.

At quarter past six, he got out of bed, leaving his sons to sleep, and rang Mr James Monahan, a solicitor at Michael Daley's law firm in Maroubra, a seaside suburb of Sydney.

'Jim, I'm in terrible trouble. There's been a shooting.'

'I'll meet you at Michael's at 8 o'clock.'

David repeated himself. 'There's been... I'm in terrible trouble... there's been a shooting and I want to give myself up to the police.'

Monahan then repeated his instruction. 'I'll meet you at 8 o'clock.'

A legal representative, Barry Bunton, was nominated from the law firm, and at midday, David McGregor gave himself up to police at Maroubra police station. He was accompanied by Barry Bunton, who was present when he underwent an ERISP (Electronically Recorded Interview of a Suspected Person).

The interviewing officer was Detective Sergeant Joe Cassar, and he was accompanied by Detective Senior Constable Lindsay Kerfoot. The interview commenced at 1.23 pm and went on until 8.44 pm. It was a very long interview even allowing for the usual breaks. David McGregor told the two detectives all about trials and tribulations which had led up to the shooting, and the medication he used to manage his stress was discussed at some length. He told them he'd been prescribed Zoloft and the last time he'd taken it had been two weeks previously, the day before he'd gone to Tamworth for a family court hearing. He hadn't intended that to be the last time, but he'd forgotten to take his medication with him, so he couldn't take it, and when he'd got back home, he'd felt much better without it and so hadn't bothered with it since. However, that contradicted what he'd said earlier in the interview when he'd said he'd been prescribed Zoloft, had taken them for a month and had felt better, although he didn't know whether that had been as a result of the medication or just because he'd felt stronger, but whatever the reason for his feeling better, he'd thrown the tablets away after a month. He confirmed the dosage as being one hundred milligrams per day and that he'd been taking it for a period of three months. When asked what effect it had had on him, he said it had made him feel like a zombie, in that it was like having a hangover and not being able to think as clearly he wanted to.

David McGregor was formally charged with the murder of his former de facto wife, thirty-nine-year-old Vivian Lillias Acheson, and appeared at Waverley Local Court. No fact sheet was tendered to the court, with Magistrate Caroline Barkell ordering the case to be transferred to Armidale Local Court for mention on 6 January 2003. McGregor's lawyer appealed for medical attention, asking for him to be treated for his high blood pressure and depression. This request was granted and he was remanded in custody.

Bail wasn't sought, and he was instructed to face a committal hearing the following month, on 19 February, when the magistrate considered the evidence in the case.

Solicitor Clayton Croft appeared on 22 April for a brief hearing on McGregor's behalf, and the matter eventually went before the Supreme Court, with the trial starting on Monday, 24 May 2004, at Armidale.

The jury was empanelled and police witnesses called, although it wasn't until Wednesday, 4 June, 2004 that the jury heard McGregor speak for the first time, when they viewed the lengthy seven-hour statement he'd made at Maroubra police station on Monday, 9 December, 2002, in which he described the events leading up to the shooting, what he did after and before he gave himself up, the distress he'd been caused by the custody battle and his medication.

I was present to interpret the drug dosages prescribed, in particular that of Zoloft, to determine how much McGregor would or would not have been affected at the time of the tragedy. I initially gave some background to the use of the drug and listed some of its adverse side effects, including dizziness, nausea, fatigue and somnolence (sleepiness). However, I said that I thought that once a patient had been stabilised to the drug, those undesirable side effects would be minimal. In conclusion, I said, 'I am of the opinion that at the time of the incident Goebel McGregor was not affected by the medication

Zoloft (sertraline), as the drug was allegedly discontinued two weeks earlier, and would no longer be present in his blood.'

The trial lasted almost two weeks and, by a majority verdict, the jury found David McGregor guilty of murdering Vivian Acheson, rejecting the argument that the shooting had been provocative defence. He was sentenced to a maximum of twenty years, with a non-parole period of fifteen years. With time in custody, he would be eligible for parole in December 2017.

The couple's two young sons were the real losers from this case, because with neither parent able to take care of them, they were placed in the care of the Department of Community Services.

If David McGregor had kept taking his prescribed medication, he may have been able to resist the taunts of his former de facto, and maybe this story would have had a very different outcome, or indeed, it may never have even been written.

24

A Coach, a Hooker and a Hit of 'Meth' - with a Hint of Heroin

'Experience is a hard teacher because she gives the test first, the lesson afterwards'

~ Veron Sanders Law

Born on 22 July 1963, Ian Avenel Gray loved his football (soccer) with a passion. He grew up in Manly Vale, a delightful seaside suburb of northern Sydney, and began playing soccer at Manly Vale Soccer Club and Western Suburbs SC (NSW), moving on later to APIA (Associazione Poli-sportiva Italo Australiana) Leichhardt Tigers Football Club, a semi-professional soccer club based in the Sydney suburb of Leichhardt. The club was formed in 1954 as APIA Leichhardt by Italian Australians, and Gray played for them for five seasons and eighty-five games before signing for Marconi, for whom he played for seven seasons and over a hundred and fifty games, in the process winning three titles, the last as captain in 1993.

As an experienced defender or midfielder, his career also saw him represent Australia thirty-five times from 1981 to 1992, and in 2004, he was not only inducted into the Australian Football (Soccer) Hall of Fame (Award of Distinction), but also became a member of the Football Federation Australia Appeals committee.

He retired from professional football in 1995, but continued to play at an amateur level for the Maccabi Masters and Team Bondi while also coaching junior players at the Maccabi Hakoah Football Club in the Under 15 State Youth League. He was an excellent coach, mentoring a number of players during their early years, and earned the affectionate moniker of Iggy.

However, his life was to take a fatal turn in 2008 when he took a working holiday in Phuket, Thailand. One night, he got caught up in a bar argument, and while he was waiting for a taxi, he was set upon and attacked with an iron bar, resulting in serious head injuries. It was an attack from which he never fully recovered, yet he hung in there and continued to mentor young soccer players even though he no longer felt a hundred per cent.

It therefore came as a great surprise when he failed to show for the training session of a junior team at 5 pm on 15 February 2010. It was so out of character that both club officials and the boys became very worried. Telephone calls, which became ever more frantic, were made, but each one met with no response, so some of his friends decided to go to his apartment on Onslow Ave, Elizabeth Bay to investigate. When they arrived at 10.45 pm, they could hear the sound of Gray's television, but knocking on the door and ringing the bell didn't garner any response, so they elected to force an entry.

They found Gray sitting on a sofa in the lounge room. He was dead.

He was wearing a pair of shorts with a small towel on his chest. A small puncture mark on the inside of his right arm, consistent with a track mark, was also noted, as was some ominous white foam on his nostrils. Police were promptly called, followed by an ambulance. A crime scene was set up and specialist forensic officers and detectives from Kings Cross carried out examinations and collected potential exhibits. A quantity of drug paraphernalia, which included a spoon and several swabs lay near Gray's body, and a used syringe was found in the kitchen bin. The scene bore all the hallmarks of a drug overdose.

Gray's body was taken to the Glebe Department of Forensic Medicine the following morning, and the post-mortem was carried out by Dr Rianie Janse Van Vuuren at 9 am on 17 February 2010. The examination showed an enlarged heart with mild coronary atherosclerosis. There was oedema fluid in the trachea and bronchi, and the lungs were congested and oedematous. There was also emphysematous change and a white foam plume on his nostrils.

Such symptoms are typical of a polydrug overdosage by central nervous system (CNS) depressants and CNS stimulants.

That was borne out by the subsequent toxicology report, which revealed that a blood sample taken from Gray at the post-mortem contained:

- benzoylecgonine 0.24 milligrams per litre,
- methylamphetamine 0.12 milligrams per litre,
- amphetamine less than 0.03 milligrams per litre,
- morphine (free) 0.06 milligrams per litre,
- codeine (free) less than 0.05 milligrams per litre,
- phentermine 0.23 milligrams per litre,
- naproxen 0.9 milligrams per litre, and
- citalopram 0.1 milligrams per litre.

A urine sample showed up methylamphetamine, amphetamine, citalopram, phentermine, levamisole, monoacetylmorphine and acetylcodeine, while a nasal swab revealed the presence of cocaine, which accounted for the detection of benzoylecgonine in his blood.

I concluded that the levels of methylamphetamine and phentermine, together with morphine, in Ian Avenel Gray's blood, were consistent with the combined effect of these drugs, resulting in his death. Given the presence of monoacetylmorphine and acetylcodeine (an impurity in street-grade heroin) in his urine, it's likely that some, if not all, of the morphine had been derived from heroin ingestion.

As sad as Gray's passing was, everyone wanted to know how the tragedy had happened. His close friends were puzzled and confused, as they all said that Gray had loathed drugs, and they found it impossible to believe that he'd been leading a double life, but unfortunately, that is exactly what he appeared to have been doing.

It's something that happens quite often to people who have been subjected to a trauma that isn't properly treated. As a way to escape and to relieve the psychological and/or physical pain endured, they take to substance abuse. Gray's father said he'd never fully recovered from the violent attack in Thailand, which had left him with severe head injuries, resulting in some apparent temporary paralysis and a brain injury. Subsequently, he'd suffered memory loss, along with some personality changes and depression.

His situation peaked on Sunday, 14 February, 2010, when at 5 am, he asked his flatmate and friend, Belynda Adamou, to accompany him to Darlinghurst Road, Darlinghurst, Sydney, where they met up with an attractive twenty-two-year-old woman, Sherryn Marie Davis, who was employed as an escort at Porky's nightclub. She accompanied Gray back to his unit, without Belynda, although she later spoke to Gray on her mobile phone, when he told her he was with Sherryn.

Later that same morning, Gray gave Sherryn a hundred and fifty dollars to buy him some ice (a potent form of methylamphetamine), and arranged to meet her again that evening. Meanwhile, he went off to soccer training and watched an A-league game at the Sydney Football Stadium between Sydney FC and Melbourne Victory. While he was doing that, Sherryn bought some heroin for herself some ice for him. They then met up as planned.

Belynda returned to the unit late in the evening and found Gray in the lounge, slumped in a chair. He was having difficulty breathing, as he was gurgling from his mouth. Sherryn was standing beside him, holding a small towel around his arm like a tourniquet. Two fresh syringes, a spoon, water and swabs lay nearby. She turned to Belynda and said, 'I just shot him up. He said he'd had heroin before'.

'Will he be okay?' Belynda asked

'Yeah,' Sherryn replied. 'He'll be alright.'

Knowing that Gray had a history of drug use (he'd smoked methylamphetamine and used cocaine, ecstasy and heroin), Belynda took her leave, reassuring herself that everything would be fine.

However, one or two doubts niggled away at the back of her mind, so the following morning, she contacted Sherryn at about 9 am to check on his wellbeing. Sherryn told her that Gray was okay.

In the meantime, Gray's wallet, iPhone and a number of other personal items went missing.

Police investigations and a tip-off led to Sherryn Davis' arrest at Porky's, and she was taken into custody and subsequently charged with the manslaughter of Ian Gray, supplying a prohibited drug and stealing from him goods worth an estimated $3,000, including a laptop, some clothing and a digital camera. She didn't apply for bail at the Central Local Court, although it was formally refused anyway, and even more curiously, she didn't come up from her cell to appear before court.

On 27 May 2010, she appeared before Justice Antony Townsden at Sydney Central Local Court both to answer the charges. The earlier manslaughter charge had been withdrawn the previous month after it had been revealed at an inquest that the former soccer star had had a plethora of drugs in his system. The stimulants, methylamphetamine, cocaine and phentermine together would have increased Gray's blood pressure markedly and placed some strain on his heart, and the hit of heroin by itself would not have been sufficient to tip him over the edge.

While in custody, Sherryn Davis had written to Gray's parents, expressing her sorrow and contrition. She wrote, 'Although I only met your son briefly for that evening, I never wished this upon him nor did I ever mean 4 (for) this to happen. I think about my actions daily and find it hard to forgive myself.

'I spent the evening with your son only to find that he had passed away sometime during the night while I was asleep in his bed. I was scared and in shock to find your son the way he was. I fled the premises taking various items which were not mine and I regret doing so.'

By the time of the court hearing, she was five months pregnant, although the paternity of the unborn child wasn't made known, and she pleaded guilty to supplying Gray with heroin on 14 February and to larceny, admitting that she took $3000 worth of his property.

Mr Aj David Karim, who appeared on her behalf, told the magistrate that she had a 'significant amount of remorse and contrition'. He also said that she had been under the influence of a significant number of drugs at the time, and that 'putting the issue of morality aside, it [the larceny] is an offence which was opportunistic, where there was no planning'. By way of mitigation, he added that Sherryn had had a difficult childhood, living between foster homes, before becoming a sex worker at fourteen and a heroin addict at an age when 'most other children were watching *Home and Away*'.

In passing sentence, Justice Townsden took all that into account and placed her on a two-year good behaviour bond, which meant she got off very lightly, given that she'd been charged with manslaughter (though later withdrawn), supplying a prohibited drug and stealing property.

Hundreds of mourners – including other Socceroos, Mark Bosnich, Roddie Slater and Steve Corica – attended Gray's funeral to pay their respects. Members of the Maccabi Under-15s acted as ushers.

In a packed Salvation Army church, an emotional former Socceroos captain Tony Henderson paid tribute to his former teammate saying, 'I'm sick of the rubbish that gets written [in the newspapers] about this guy. All I know is, that's Ian Gray. I'm not interested in anything else anyone's got to say. That's the bottom line. He's gone and the hole will never be filled'.

His sister, Yvonne, described how Gray had had a strong work ethic installed in him by his father, who had been the driving force in his professional life. To illustrate the point, she recounted a story where Ian asked his father for a puppy. His father replied that he could have the puppy if he became captain and top scorer for the NSW football team. Taking up the challenge, he did. She concluded, 'I know he would have been amazed and humbled by the number of people that have come today'.

Mr Andy Harper, a former National Soccer League player and now a Fox Sports presenter, told the gathering, 'In a world beset by selfishness he was selfless. To him the team was everything. We all loved playing with you, playing for you. Our captain, be still, at rest'.

It's an unfortunate trait of humans to resort to substance abuse to try to relieve stress brought about by overwork and/or health issues, but that's exactly what Gray did. The inquest found that his was an accidental death, but in a fitting tribute, as he looked out over the funeral crowd packed with youngsters, Mark Bosnich said, 'Someone like Ian Gray, you don't replace. The thing that stood out from his service was the number of kids here. He's left a legacy'.

25
Butchery and Body Parts: The Murder of Nicole Grant

'I went to the laundry and got a power saw and dismembered her body because I was initially just going to dispose of the body, but fearful of being seen taking the body out of the unit.'
~ *Neal Richardson*

Gerringong is a quaint seaside village on the south coast of New South Wales. Set against a backdrop of Seven Mile Beach National Park, with great surfing at Werri Beach, it's a haven of peace and calm, making it a delightful tourist destination.

On the morning of 30 September 2010, a local man working on a locked gate at the end of Sims Road noticed a bed sheet flapping in the breeze near a lantana bush. Upon closer inspection, he saw three orange plastic garbage bags underneath. As he drew closer, a putrid smell assaulted his senses and he noticed decomposing flesh and bone in one of the ruptured bags. Thinking it could be something sinister, he contacted the local police who arrived a short time later, together with forensic personnel and detectives, to inspect the malodorous packages.

Initially, it was thought the remains were possibly of animal origin and that some unsociable person had left the waste material under the roadside bushes. A presumptive test carried out on the blood-stained bed sheet returned a negative test for human blood, while a local veterinarian who inspected the contents of one of the bags identified one of the bones to be an animal pelvis, probably that of a young calf. However, there was some doubt about the other contents.

Later that afternoon, police contacted the Glebe mortuary and spoke to the duty pathologist, Dr Istvan Szentmariay, regarding the find. He requested that some photographs be sent for review. Unfortunately, they were sent via email, and were of such low quality, he was unable to ascertain whether the remains were human or non-human. Consequently, he asked for the specimens to be taken to the mortuary for a closer examination, which confirmed they were, in fact, human. A portion of a left hand was found in a condition that still enabled fingerprints to be taken, thus making it possible to identify the victim. The poor person in question was Nicole Kirrilee Grant, a prostitute known to the police. The submitted exhibits were truly a potpourri, with both animal and human remains being present. Multiple plastic bags of different types contained human remains in various stages of decomposition; some were dried and others were moist. The skeletal remains showed the presence of multiple cuts on various bones, including the left and right clavicle, left and right scapula, multiple ribs, bones of both arms, bones of both legs, and the thoracic and lumbar vertebrae. A black bag containing a GMC brand power saw with human material and bone in the teeth was also present, along with a decomposing woman's head. Nicole's body had been extensively butchered prior to disposal.

Her body parts arrived at the Glebe Department of Forensic Medicine on the morning of 1 October, 2010, and the post-mortem was carried out by Dr Istvan Szentmariay on 4 and 5 October, 2010.

The entire exhibit, consisting of multiple body parts, was x-rayed, but no suspicious radio-opaque material, such as a bullet, was observed. The report on the decomposing human torso made for grim reading, and I've reproduced some of it here so you can gain some idea of the horror.

The body parts were moist, with slippery surfaces and extensive adiopocere formation. Most of the remaining skin was relatively well preserved and showed normal colour. Posteriorly, the skin covered the torso to the level of the lower neck, on both sides to the level of the armpits. On the right side the skin was recognisable down to the level of the 9th rib and on the left side at around the 12th rib. Slightly above this level was a nearly vertical full thickness slit-like defect which measured 4.6 cm in length; no definite underlying wound track was identified. There was a large linear full thickness skin defect connecting the right – anterior-lower neck area to the lateral aspect of the right breast (gaping defect). The inferior border of the skin still present was the lower third of the right breast and about 10 cm below the inferior level of the left breast.

A large portion of the skin of the left breast was not present (nipples could not be identified), leaving an irregularly oval shaped defect in this area, measuring up to 16 cm in largest dimension. There were three vertically arranged (on top of each other) slightly gaping defects on the superior aspect of the left breast. The underlying soft tissue was soft and decomposing; no definite wound tracks were identified. In all the described parts of the torso, the skin margins were soft, thinned and were decomposing.

As for the other decomposing body parts, Dr Szentmariay reported: 'Decomposing head with an attached off-white/light grey empty collapsed plastic bag along with occasional small pieces of soft tissue. The remaining relatively small amount of brain material inside the skull was in a semi liquid state; no material reminiscent of blood was noted. The content of the cranial cavity was visible through the foramen magnum. The overall weight of the specimen was 2700 g. Due to post-mortem decompositional changes, a portion of the right side of the scalp was nearly completely separated and measured 25.5 x 29 cm (flattened) with some hair still present on it (sampled and taken by police for colour and length – identification). Three small piercing holes were noted in the right earlobe. The soft tissue removed from the head weighed

660 g. The peeled, seemingly blonde hair weighed 480 g and it measured up to 25-30 cm in length'.

However, he also noted that the post-mortem examination had, 'a somewhat limited value due to decompositional changes, certain tissues were not recovered and no forensically important major neck structures could be evaluated for possible injuries. There were numerous skin defects which may represent in vivo (sustained while alive) injuries along multiple defects on the anterior aspect of the liver however exact interpretation of these lesions can be difficult. Similarly, defects described above involving the anterior/inferior aspect of the liver may have been inflicted. The injury pattern of some vertebrae (cuts) suggests infliction from the front (rather than from the back). The presence of multiple blade marks on the face is rather unusual in dismemberment cases. Some cuts were described as only 1 mm in width and some as much as 6 mm, which may be a reflection of the sharp instrument(s) used'.

The toxicology report revealed that a liver sample (a suitable blood sample was not available) taken at the post-mortem was found to have present codeine 0.37 milligrams per kilogram. No other drugs were detected.

The reported drug concentrations in liver from codeine fatalities range from 0.6 to 45 mg/kg, with an average being 6.8 mg/kg. The level of the drug detected in Nicole Grant's liver (0.37 mg/kg) was far short of a fatal concentration and indicated that the drug had been ingested sometime earlier prior to death. I concluded that, 'the level of codeine detected in Ms Nicole Grant's liver is consistent with a moderate ingestion of the drug sometime before her death'.

Abusive people are often very dependent upon their partners for their sense of self-esteem. While appearing to be powerful, they often feel powerless within themselves and their relationship may be the only place where they have a sense of power. By keeping their partners in a diminished, fearful or dependent state, they try to ensure that their partners are kept under control. Unfortunately for Nicole, she'd been drawn into a violent, abusive relationship with such a person namely, Neal Richardson.

They shared a unit in Malabar, in the east of Sydney, and had an 'on and off' relationship. Their lifestyle was unusual, with Nicole working as a prostitute to supplement a pension, and their relationship was characterised by drug and alcohol abuse. But worse than that was the physical abuse that that led to.

It peaked after Nicole made a statement to a Maroubra police officer on 23 October, 2009 while she was in the Prince of Wales Hospital. She said that Richardson had assaulted her with a car lock, causing the severe injuries that she had, and that previously, he'd said he'd had enough of her and had grabbed her around the neck with a tartan scarf and dragged her by her leg before binding her with cable ties. At the same time, he'd shouted at her, 'that's why your sister died, you're both c★★ts. [Nicole's twin sister had been murdered some years earlier in Brisbane.] Shut up, shut up. I don't want to hear you cry, this will stop you from crying'. Then he'd stuffed a sock down her throat and covered her mouth with masking tape before kneeing her in the chest and stomach. When he'd eventually fallen asleep, she'd been able to free herself by using a cigarette lighter to burn the cable ties.

She also told the police, 'I'm terrified of Neal and I don't want to go back to the unit'. Then she asked for emergency accommodation.

Richardson was subsequently charged with assaulting her, occasioning her actual bodily harm, in October 2009, and she was due to give evidence against him the following year, on 19 April 2010.

Unfortunately, in the meantime, she returned to the unit that she and Richardson shared, and faced further physical and mental abuse.

Shortly after midnight on 18 April, the day before she was due to give evidence against Richardson, Nicole made a number of calls to the National Australia Bank, requesting a new credit card. She appeared to be distressed.

The following day, Richardson, who had been on remand for a month after the assault charge, duly turned up at Waverly Local Court, but Nicole didn't, and the assault charge against him was dismissed. Later that same day, Richardson was observed purchasing three orange plastic bags and a shovel, and that evening, a neighbour saw him beside his car with a removalist-type trolley, the latter two items being found later by police in the boot of Richardson's car, both with blood stains that matched Nicole's DNA. Nicole was never seen alive again.

Following the discovery of Nicole's body parts in three orange plastic sacks, detectives and forensics went to work with a passion and gathered enough evidence to have Neal Richardson arrested. The matter then went before Justice Lucy McCullum in the NSW Supreme Court, Kings Street, Sydney, on 1 November 2011.

The crown prosecutor, Sarah Huggett, started by alleging that Neal Richardson, 45, had murdered Nicole Grant, 41, between 17 and 25 April, 2010, before dismembering her body and placing the body parts into plastic garbage bags and dumping them into a paddock.

Detective Phillip Brown said he'd gone to the Gerringong property on 30 September 2010 after a neighbour had contacted the police. On arrival, he'd seen an orange bag under a large bush. The bag had contained what appeared to be a pelvis bone and a smaller black bag, which on further investigation had been found to be concealing a GMC brand power saw covered in what looked like human material and bone debris. The bag had also held a decomposing woman's head.

A crime scene officer, Mark Hollands, also provided testimony regarding the exhibits found on the Gerringong property.

Graham Turnbull, SC, appearing for Neal Richardson, admitted that his client, 'did cut up the body of Nicole Kirrilee Grant and dispose of it'. But he pointed out that not only could the Crown not prove Richardson had caused her death, but that Nicole Grant had been a 'sick woman', with psychiatric problems who had been working as a prostitute for many years, and had abused alcohol and drugs.

Sarah Huggett said that although the Crown could not point to the precise cause of the death of Nicola, Richardson had earlier been charged with assaulting her, occasioning her actual bodily harm, in October 2009, and that she'd been due to give evidence against him on 19 April, 2010. She continued, saying that shortly after midnight on 18 April, Nicola had made calls, parts of which had been recorded, asking for a new key card from the National Australia Bank. 'Ms Grant sounds, at times, incoherent. That may have been because she had taken drugs or alcohol, but she could also be heard crying and in distress.'

The court heard that Richardson had also spoken to the operator, and in contrast to Nicola, had been quite calm, politely providing all the necessary information. A neighbour who had lent them her mobile phone to make the call to the bank recalled that when the phone had been returned, Nicola had 'a bloody mouth'.

The prosecutor said, 'That was the last time the deceased was seen or heard of alive'.

Graham Turnbull told the jury that Nicola's twin sister had been murdered in 1991, in Brisbane, and that had affected some of the things she'd told the police and other people. He said that through her alcohol, drug use and psychiatric condition, 'Ms Grant became someone who was explosive, belligerent, hard to handle, unreasonable and self-destructive.'

When questioned, Neal Richardson admitted using a power saw to dismember Nicole's body, but said it was after she'd fallen and fatally hit her head on a coffee table. He said that she'd been 'extremely intoxicated' after taking some tablets and had wanted to return to Kings Cross, but that he'd tried to stop her. He explained that she'd started to hit him, trying to get past to the front door, but 'I pushed her hands away from me. We both fell over and she smashed her head on the coffee table in the lounge room and she remained on the floor and she didn't move'.

He then said the sight of his girlfriend lying on the floor had caused him to become distraught and panic because of the recent assault charge against him, so he'd taken Nicole's body into the bathroom. He carried on, 'I went to the laundry and got a power saw and dismembered her body, because I was initially just going to dispose of the body, but I was fearful of being seen taking the body out of the unit'. He said that he'd started on her feet and worked his way up, cutting off pieces that would fit into the garbage bags.

Graham Turnbull asked him if he could 'still see' what he'd done.

Richardson replied, 'I see it every day, several times a day. That image is instilled in my mind'.

Turnbull then asked him if he'd killed Nicola to stop her from going to court.

'No,' came the answer. 'She never had any intention of going to court.'

Richardson also told the court that Nicola had told him that her sister had been murdered in Brisbane, in 1991, and that her head had been half severed, she'd had cable ties around her hands, wire around her body and had been burned from the waist down. He said, 'She wanted me to kill her in a similar way her sister was murdered'.

Richardson was then cross-examined by Sarah Huggett regarding the dismemberment of Nicola's body. She suggested that he'd cut up her body to 'hide or disguise injuries he had inflicted on her'.

He replied that the only reason he'd cut up her body was 'to make it as small as I possibly could to fit into the garbage bags'.

However, other evidence provided by the pathologist revealed that the dismemberment had been extensive, with not only her body being cut to pieces, but her hands and even the nipples from her breasts being removed before being placed into the garbage bags. The bags had been dumped under a lantana bush because Richardson had found the ground too hard to dig.

Regarding the previous assault charge, Richardson denied influencing Nicole to not give evidence against him, telling the jury she'd told him several times she wouldn't attend.

Sarah Huggett asked, 'You didn't want to go back to jail on Monday?'

Richardson answered, 'I never once thought I was. I had no fear of that court case,'

Sarah Huggett repeated the question. 'You didn't want to go back to jail on Monday, 19?'

'Of course not.'

Richardson agreed he'd lied to the police and others about Nicola's whereabouts, saying she'd run off with a rich man from Blacktown, in order to protect himself. 'I was going to lie to every single person.'

Sarah Huggett retorted, 'I suggest you are continuing to lie in the witness box'.

'No, I'm not,' Richardson replied.

After some further discussion, the jury retired to consider their verdict. It had been three long weeks, but they needed less than two full days of deliberation to find Richardson guilty of murder by a majority verdict.

The court found that Richardson had been partly motivated to cut up Nicole's body to remove evidence of injuries he'd inflicted upon her. Justice Lucy McCullum, rejecting the argument that Nicole's body had been dismembered for transport purposes only, said, 'Some of the parts had been cut into smaller pieces than can sensibly be explained, one foot was cut in two, a little finger and both nipples had been removed, reflecting a higher level of criminality'.

She also noted that the jury had rejected his claim that Nicole had died hitting her head on a coffee table after falling during a fight.

Turning to the mater of the phone calls to the bank, Justice McCallum found that it had been Richardson's intention to kill Nicole and that he'd forced her to make calls to the bank so he would have access to her bank account after her death. She commented, 'The recordings of those telephone calls are chilling. They reveal that Ms Grant was at times incoherent, angry, frustrated and distressed. The offender, by contrast, was calm, politely providing the information required by the bank'.

Richardson was sentenced to a maximum of twenty-eight years, with a non-parole period of twenty-one years.

But it wasn't quite over.

The following year, on 17 September 2013, Neal Richardson's lawyers appeared in the NSW Court of Criminal Appeal to argue against both his conviction and the sentence. Central to the appeal was the statement made by Nicola Grant to police in October, 2009 and shown to the jury during the trial, in which she alleged Richardson had tied her up with cable ties, gagged and assaulted her.

Richardson's barrister, Nicole Carroll, from George Sten & Co, told the Appeal Court that the jury should not have heard about Richardson's previous assault on Nicole because it 'would amount to a miscarriage of justice'.

But the appeal judge, Justice Megan Latham, responded by saying that the trial judge, Lucy McCallum, had delivered a direction to jurors regarding the statement of evidence of violent tendencies of Richardson before they'd made their decision.

Also on the panel, Chief Judge at Common Law, Clifton Hoeben, said that the defence council at the trial hadn't objected to the statement being shown to the jury and had used it to support Richardson's explanation as to why he'd disposed of Nicole's body the way he had because he was sure 'police would believe I killed her'.

Barrister Nicole Carroll also argued that too much weight had been placed on the dismemberment of Nicole's body, resulting in a 'manifestly excessive' sentence, but Justice Clifton Hoeben commented, 'The point of distinction which the appellant sought to draw between the treatment of the deceased's corpse after death being a matter of aggravation rather than going to the seriousness of the offence, is a distinction without a difference'.

Justice Latham was even more critical, saying, 'This was, in my view, a completely unmeritorious appeal. Unfortunately, the maintenance of such appeals in this jurisdiction inevitably delays the listing of other conviction appeals with real prospects of success'.

The three appeals Judges then dismissed the appeal, saying that the previous assault had been a relevant motive because Nicole Grant had been killed before she'd been due to give evidence about the offence.

With time in custody, Neal Richardson will be eligible for parole in May 2031.

26 Almost a Murder: The 'Romeo and Juliet' Case

'For never was a story of more woe than this
of Juliet and her Romeo.'
~ William Shakespeare, Romeo and Juliet

Samantha Holland and Joel Betts shared an apartment in Chippendale, an inner Sydney suburb, and from the outside, they seemed to be the perfect couple. They were both well educated, pleasing on the eye - Samantha with her blonde hair and sparkling blue eyes, and Joel with his rugged, handsome, dark looks - and held down good jobs - Samantha worked as a mobile sales coordinator, while Joel had a promising future running his own communication business, having previously had a stint as a presenter on Foxtel.

But behind the everyday facade, all was not what it seemed.

Joel was born and raised in Sydney, NSW. His parents separated when he was six, and he only saw his father once after the age of ten. He had a good relationship with both his mother, who worked as a medical receptionist, and brother. The family problems began when he was eight years old, around the time his mother met a builder called Walter. They got married and had two daughters, but Walter was a very violent man, and on one occasion, he stabbed Joel's mother and the police became involved. As frequently happens, she chose to stay with him even though he was violent to her and Joel.

It's impossible to know with any degree of certainty what goes on behind closed doors, but emotional abuse and domestic violence leave their marks, both mentally and physically. In spite of the abuse, Joel managed to graduate from high school in 1997, going on to Macquarie University, where he gained a bachelor's degree in commerce in 2001. He later appeared on Australian Survivor for thirty-eight days.

His first relationship was with a young woman, Claudia, whom he met at high school. It lasted seven years, during which time she provided constant emotional support by coaching and encouraging him so much that she 'felt like the mother'. However, it couldn't go on, as it was wearing her out, and the relationship became an on-off affair before they finally called it a day. Every relationship has its ups and downs, but that one, with its constant support, was pivotal to Joel's life, and the break-up impacted upon future relationships – and lives.

In December 2007, Joel started dating Samantha Holland. At the time, they were both studying for degrees at Sydney University: Joel, a Masters in Cross-Cultural Communication and Samantha, a Bachelor of Liberal Studies. Joel was living in Kirribilli and Samantha in Camperdown. Finances were rather tight, so he took up Samantha's offer and moved into her unit, which she shared with three others. After a few months, he moved out and shared a flat in Randwick with Kate Roberts.

Nearly two years later, in October 2009, Joel and Samantha, feeling that the bond between them was now solid, decided to rent one of the Waldorf Apartments in Chippen Street, Chippendale, and for a time, they shared good times and were happy. Then, on Thursday, 25 March, just five months later, after a lengthy discussion about their relationship, Samantha decided to call it quits.

She called her mother in the early hours of 26 March to give her the news and ask her to pick her up. Early the following morning, she left with a suitcase of clothes and went to stay with her family, who lived in North Richmond.

She remained in contact with Joel, with both of them bobbing up and down on the opposite ends of an emotional see-saw, although she did say to him, 'I don't know why we're both fighting so hard for something that is clearly already over'.

After a few more days, thinking the matter had been settled, Samantha set out to find suitable accommodation, moving into a house shared by Kate Mann and Tom Roth. On 9 April, Joel called her to let her know that he would be moving out of the Waldorf apartment on the weekend of 17–18 April.

'I'm organising a truck to take my things into storage next weekend. Let me know if you want me to take any of your stuff anywhere.'

'I don't think it's a good idea that we're there at the same time,' Samantha replied, 'so if you can tell me exactly when you'll be moving your stuff, I can organise to move mine at a different time. I won't need to use the truck because my family has offered to help me out'.

She confirmed the arrangement the following week so as to be sure of the time when Joel wouldn't be there.

Joel said, 'I'm moving my stuff on Sunday [18 April]'.

'That's fine,' Samantha replied. 'I'll move my stuff on Saturday then. What time will you be leaving the apartment?'

'I have a work function to go to by 10.30 am, so I'll be gone by then.'

'Okay, I'll get there after 10.30 am. What time will you be back?'

'No worries, I can be gone all day if you'll be at the apartment.'

In the week leading up to the weekend, Joel rang her again, this time asking whether she'd like a coffee. He wanted them to get back together and was anxious to talk to her and tell her how well they worked together. She agreed to meet him at a café, where they discussed various things, including her graduation at Sydney University. Inevitably, the conversation turned back to their relationship. Joel expressed his disbelief at the reason they'd broken up, but Samantha made it clear she had no intention of sharing him with another woman, as she didn't 'want to have a threesome'.

Just before they left the café, Samantha said, 'The question I asked in the café was obvious. Did you or did you not sleep with other people? You were deliberately manipulating my emotions and reactions by leaving out that information (that you slept with her). The fact that you went so far as to tell me superfluous information ... like you slept on a blow-up mattress at Michelle's place ... is also an indication that you knew whether or not you had sex. That girl was an important part of the conversation, but you failed to mention that you had slept with her'.

'I haven't done anything wrong', Joel blustered.

'You haven't done anything wrong,' Samantha retorted, 'but it puts all the other shit you were saying into perspective. Thank you for the tea, goodbye, and have a nice night'.

From that point on, Samantha decided not to respond to any contact or communication from him. However, undeterred, he kept calling - several times a day, every day, up until 16 April - and she kept ignoring him.

On the morning of Saturday, 17 April, Samantha met up with her friends and had breakfast at an east Sydney café. Her housemate, Kate Mann, then drove her to the Waldorf apartment. It was just after 11 am. She was going to pack up her possessions and had arranged for her brother, Todd, to call around and help her move them. She took her swipe key from her handbag, nodded to the women at the front desk and rode the lift to third floor. As she pushed the apartment door open, Joel walked out of the bedroom. He hadn't stuck to the agreement.

'You weren't meant to be here,' Samantha said, her voice conveying her annoyance.

As she put her handbag down on the kitchen bench, Joel responded, 'I've been trying to contact you. I want to talk to you'.

'I know. I'm not interested in listening.'

At 12.10 pm, her brother texted to let her know he'd arrived at the apartment block. *I'm here. Where should I park?*

Samantha texted back. *On the street.*

At 12.23 pm, she texted again. *Give me a couple of minutes. Joel is here. Sorry.*

That was her last authentic text.

Joel then attempted to talk her into forgiving him and resuming their relationship, only for her to remind him how he'd had multiple dates with other young women and had 'had weird stuff with a girl from Lebanon'.

'What happened with Yaara was wrong by you. Can't you try and understand this from my perspective?'

'I've been trying very hard for the past eighteen months to understand this from your perspective,' Samantha replied, 'and that's the only reason I'm still here. And now I'm done. The damage to our relationship has been done'.

Similar exchanges went on for some time, with Joel trying to hug Samantha on a number of occasions. Then she remembered that her brother was waiting downstairs and started to rummage through her handbag for the swipe key so she could go and let him in.

'I'm done,' she said. 'And as always, it's me that has to show the strength of my convictions, to say something and stick by it. You can't expect to tell me yes-no-yes-no and for me to be here through all of it. I'm done, it's over. I'm going downstairs to let Todd in.'

As she stepped towards the door, Joel barred her way.

'Let me past.'

Joel moved to one side, but as she turned the handle, he started stabbing her with a short vegetable knife, raining blows down on her back. Samantha spun around and started screaming, long repeated screams, but Joel continued stabbing her. As they fell to the floor, he stabbed her shoulders and the right side of her neck.

Shocked and terrified, Samantha picked herself up and ran towards the kitchen, reaching over the preparation surface to pick up her mobile phone. Joel pulled her back, grabbed the phone out of her hands and threw it across the room. He then started stabbing her in the neck. Samantha made another attempt to escape via the front door, but was thwarted again. Joel put the knife to his wrist and cut it. Then he dropped to his knees, stabbing himself in the neck before turning his attention to Samantha for a further attack.

She screamed, 'You're going to gaol. Todd's downstairs and he'll know it was you'.

Kneeling by the front door, Joel said, 'We'll die here together. Then we can be together for eternity'.

Samantha gasped, 'I never knew you were this fucked up'.

Joel rolled her over onto her front and started to stab her in the back again, saying, 'You're going to die'.

Samantha tried to escape a number of times, but each time, Joel managed to overpower her, and the torture continued. She tried talking to him, reasoning with him and even threatening him, but nothing worked. Bleeding and in pain, she knew she had to weaken her attacker sufficiently so she could make another last ditch effort to escape.

'If we're going to do this together,' she said, 'I should have a turn with the knife'.

She convinced Joel to give her the weapon, which she used to stab him in the stomach, but even then he still had enough strength to stop her escaping.

'Are you ready to die yet?' he asked.

He then used her mobile phone to text her brother. *We're looking like staying together. For now at least. I'll call you soon. Thanks for coming today bro. X.*

He also sent a message with an air of finality to Samantha's mother. *Mum I love you.*

It was then about 1.45 pm. Joel was weakened from his injuries, so Samantha tried another strategy to get away from him. 'There's a good quote in the last Harry Potter book *[Harry Potter and the Deathly Hallows]* about dying that I want to read to you,' she said. 'Go and get it.'

As he went to fetch the book, she made good her escape. She dashed to the sliding door that led onto the balcony, released the bolt and threw the door open. Then she shot across to the railing, swung her legs over and landed on her bottom on the second-storey balcony below.

She was covered in blood, her hair was matted and she was wearing only her underwear. She called down to a shocked couple passing by, 'Excuse me. I need your help. I've been stabbed by my boyfriend. He's still upstairs. I need you to help me'.

Some nearby workmen saw her plight and also came to the rescue, using their ladders to reach her and help her down to the pavement below. An ambulance was summoned and she was whisked away to the Royal Prince Alfred Hospital, where she underwent surgery that evening.

The police were also alerted, and they found Joel lying on the apartment floor. He, too, was admitted to the same hospital for treatment.

Samantha was found to have multiple stab wounds to her back, neck and limbs, with twenty stab wounds to her upper back and a foreign body (knife tip) in a lower back wound. She was discharged eight days later.

Joel was found to have a number of stab wounds, the most serious of which was the abdominal stab wound, necessitating surgery, during which a number of bleeding severed arteries were found and subsequently tied off. He also had several wounds to his chest and neck. He was discharged six days later and taken into custody to face court.

Prior to the matter going to trial, Samantha provided a statement which described Joel's consumption of drugs and alcohol. While the recreational use of cannabis and cocaine were mentioned, together with excessive alcohol consumption on one particular occasion, she also spoke about a drug known as DMT.

The Director of Public Prosecutions wanted to know if it could have affected Joel's behaviour and to what extent its use was relevant to the offence.

I said that, DMT is the abbreviated term for N, N-dimethyltryptamine or dimethyltryptamine, and is a short acting (half-life of 0.5-1.5 hr.) hallucinogenic indole derivative that is structurally related to serotonin (5-hydroxytryptamine), a neurotransmitter. DMT is widely distributed throughout the plant kingdom and occurs naturally in certain South American plants, for example, Mimosa sp. As a drug of abuse, DMT is commonly smoked with tobacco and/or cannabis or other plant material. Doses of 50-150 milligrams are typical. Ingestion of the drug can produce hallucinations, intense visuals, euphoria, papillary dilation and hypertension (elevated blood pressure). Because the effects of DMT can be over in as little as thirty minutes, the drug has been dubbed as the 'the businessman's lunch'.

The rapid breakdown of DMT in the body is achieved by the enzyme monoamine oxidase (MAO). However, this degradation can be inhibited by various MAO inhibitors, such as harmine, harmaline and tetrahydroharmine.

So, would Joel Betts have been affected by DMT at the time of the offence?

That was a difficult question to answer, given the absence of a blood analysis result/s. However, the effects experienced by DMT are quite short and I would have expected them to have been over before the altercation. Furthermore, the CCTV showed the victim entering the building at 11.11 am, and for approximately an hour, despite earlier agreeing to not be present at the unit, the accused was there, talking to the victim. At 12.10 pm the victim's brother texted her to say he'd arrived at the apartment block and the victim texted back a message at 12.23 pm stating that Joel was present in the apartment. It would therefore appear, if the drug had previously been in his system, that sufficient time had elapsed for any effects to have dissipated.

As to what extent it had been relevant to the offence, my answer was that it was most likely not to have had any relevance at all.

My conclusion was, 'I'm unable to provide an opinion as to whether DMT played any part in the offence that ensued. However, given the time elapsed and the rapid breakdown of the drug in the body, it would appear unlikely DMT was instrumental in the offence, even if it was ingested.'

Joel Betts pleaded guilty to wounding with intent to murder and detain for advantage, and on 27 April, 2012, he appeared before Judge Robert Toner at the Downing Centre District Court. Before a packed courtroom, Judge Toner said, 'I find that it was the offender's intention to kill Ms Holland if he could not persuade her to be with him. It was simply a matter of luck he failed'.

A handwritten note found by police at scene of the stabbings had a line from a Bon Jovi song on it: 'You know I love you, but I hate you because I could never replace you'.

The note, which had been written a week earlier, showed that the crime had been planned.

Judge Toner also said that Ms Holland had, 'acquitted herself with great courage and intelligence' by convincing her former boyfriend to give her the knife so they could die together in a Romeo and Juliet type of scenario. In sentencing Betts, Judge Toner described the offences 'as of the utmost seriousness' and sentenced him to a maximum of sixteen years, with a non-parole period of eleven years. With time in custody, he will be eligible for parole in April 2021.

In the words of the Bard:

'These violent delights have violent ends
And in their triumph die, like fire and powder
Which, as they kiss, consume.'

~ William Shakespeare, Romeo and Juliet

Fortunately, the former lover survived and was not 'consumed' in the jealous passion.

27

Woman Overboard!

'Bacchus hath drowned more men (and women) than Neptune'
~ Old English Proverb

Alcohol has not only been widely used as a social beverage for centuries, but it's also been used in association with recreational aquatic activity in many countries, including Australia. It's well known that the consumption of alcohol diminishes a person's ability to cope physically and increases risk-taking behaviour, but a lesser known effect is that exerted in a more subtle and less coincidental role that manifests itself in the occurrence of sudden unexpected deaths in many immersion accidents, particularly those involving middle-aged people.

Many unexpected drownings of adults have occurred suddenly and appeared to be inexplicable. In such cases, an otherwise healthy individual doesn't appear to struggle or surface after submersion. A subsequent post-mortem generally provides little evidence as to the cause of death other than to suggest it was by drowning. This is most likely due to the initial struggle in which the body's carbohydrate levels are used up and the presence of alcohol, even a small amount, causes a profound drop in blood glucose levels. In turn, that leads to not just weakness and confusion, but it also virtually removes the normal temperature regulating mechanisms, causing the victim's body temperature to drop very rapidly, which results in life threatening hypothermia.

A number of studies have been carried out over the years, and results show that people who partake in recreational boating with a blood alcohol level of 0.10 grams per 100 millilitres have about a ten times higher risk of death than those who have abstained beforehand. Even small amounts of alcohol can increase this risk.

While, chemically, alcohol and water do mix, water activities, such as boating, and alcohol consumption don't.

It was a warm summer evening and Sydney Harbour was awash with recreational vessels. The place was rammed with spectators, all awaiting a great night of celebration with fireworks, music and entertainment to bring in the New Year.

Mark and Anne Jones were on one of the many vessels, and having taken up their vantage point, they opened a bottle of bubbly from an ice-filled Esky. Then with a glass of wine in hand, they settled in for a night of fun and enjoyment, starting with the 9 pm family fireworks, leading up to the main event of the midnight fireworks and beyond.

During the evening, they consumed a number of bottles of wine and Mark began to feel the worse for wear, so after the final fireworks display, he said, 'I'm beat, dear. Time for bed. Are you coming?'

But Anne was still in party mode, and she replied, 'No, no, not at the moment. I'll just finish off the last of this bubbly'.

Mark yawned, at the same time noting that his wife appeared to be quite tipsy. 'Okay, okay see you shortly.'

He left the deck and headed for the bunks below. At about 2 am, he woke from a deep sleep and noticed that Anne hadn't returned to the cabin.

What's keeping her? He wondered, and made his way up back up onto the deck. But there was no one there. He searched the upper deck, and still nothing. A feeling of dread started to engulf him. After an extensive and fruitless search of the whole vessel, he decided to call the water police (Marine Area Command).

Unfortunately, there was nothing they could do at the time other than take down particulars. The following day, Anne had still not appeared, but a few days later, her body was found floating face down in Rose Bay, a few kilometres from Sydney Harbour, having been swept there by the ocean currents.

The post-mortem didn't produce any surprises, with the cause of death being 'consistent with drowning', along with a 'high range alcohol intoxication' and a 'fatty liver'. No drugs were detected. A blood sample was found to have present alcohol 0.205 grams per decilitre (100 millilitres) of blood, while a vitreous humour sample (taken from the eye), also taken at post-mortem, was found to have present alcohol 0.225 grams per decilitre (100 millilitres). That proved to be a useful toxicological sample.

The elimination rate of alcohol in man ranges from about 0.010 grams per 100 millilitres per hour to 0.025 grams per 100 millilitres per hour, with the average rate for most individuals being about 0.015 grams per 100 millilitres per hour. The difference between the alcohol content in Anne Jones' vitreous humour (0.225 gm per cent) and her blood sample (0.205 gm per cent) differed by 0.020 gm per cent, indicating that she was in the elimination phase. It also evidenced that she was a regular drinker of alcohol, a finding supported by the fatty liver.

At a blood alcohol concentration level of 0.205 grams per 100 millilitres or above, all people are likely to come under the influence of alcohol to the extent that there will be substantial impairment of their motor skills, and of their emergency reaction skills in particular. Cognitive, motor and visual functions, such as reaction skills, tracking ability, motor co-ordination, perception, judgment and decision-making skills will be substantially impaired at this blood alcohol level and above. Judgment of time and distance is also impaired by alcohol. Decision-making can be impaired as a result of altered perceptions and/or incorrect judgment. This can result in a person not recognizing a dangerous situation, thereby reducing the time available to take evasive action.

I concluded that 'the level of alcohol in [Anne Jones's] blood together with water immersion would have substantially compromised her ability to save herself in an emergency situation resulting in her death by drowning'.

It's probable that given the amount of alcohol she'd consumed, she may have been looking for a toilet. With her level of intoxication, she would have been quite unsteady on her feet and so probably stumbled and accidentally fell over the side of the vessel and drowned.

A subsequent inquest found that it was an accidental death, with the excessive consumption of alcohol being a contributing factor.

28 The Corpse in the Creek

'You must try to generate happiness within yourself.
If you aren't happy in one place,
chances are you won't be happy anyplace'
~ ***Ernie Banks***

Eastwood, a suburb of Sydney, New South Wales, is located seventeen kilometres north-west of the Sydney central business district. The area was first settled by Europeans after the arrival of the First Fleet in 1788. Today, thanks to immigration from China and Korea, Eastwood has a population largely composed of people of Asian descent, who have transformed the commercial precinct over the past two decades.

Eastwood's claim to fame is the green Granny Smith apple, which was first grown there and has since proved to be an excellent cooking apple. Every October, the streets are cordoned off for the locals to celebrate and party at the Granny Smith Festival, complete with parades, apple-baking competitions, market stalls and fireworks.

More recently, the festival has had a more Asian influence, with Chinese dragon dancers in the Grand Parade and Chinese stallholders.

Lin Lee was twenty-six years old and suffered from severe depression, a condition that was exacerbated because his girlfriend back in his homeland, to whom he was very much attached, wasn't able to come to Australia. His depression was so bad that he'd made several attempts to take his own life. However, he coped with his problems by using Seroquel - an anti-psychotic and anti-depressant drug - psychological counselling, and long walks and solitude in the bush.

One of his favourite walks was the Terry's Creek bushwalk, which is part of a trail between Eastwood and Epping train stations that follows Terry's Creek and passes through a peaceful corridor of remnant bushland consisting of Sydney blue gums, turpentines, blackbutt eucalyptus trees and Sydney red gums, some of which are estimated to be more than two hundred years old. This canopy provides an important habitat for many bird species, including parrots, owls and kookaburras, as well as possums and bats. Terry's Creek also features a waterfall; a delightful spot in which to rest and enjoy the Aussie bush. The waterfall feeds into a pool which was once a popular swimming spot, and it must have been beautiful before urban pollution encroached upon the area. Even so, water dragons and long-necked turtles are still seen swimming in the waters from time to time. The bushwalk is a pleasant escape from city life, providing an oasis of solitude in the middle of suburbia, something Lin Lee no doubt thought before being reported missing on 10 October, 2012.

Nine days later, at around 8 am, Tae Hoon Kam left his home to walk to Eastwood railway station. He went down Essex Street to the corner of Davis Street, where he began to walk across the pedestrian footbridge that leads from Essex Street through to Vimiera Road. The wooden footbridge is about ten metres long and approximately five metres above Terry's Creek. It was a warm, sunny morning and the birdlife - kookaburras and currawongs - was making its presence felt in the surrounding eucalyptus trees while half dozen ducks were feeding and making a ruckus in the stream. As Tae was crossing the bridge, he looked down into the water below and something caught his eye. Curious as to what it might be, he stopped and looked at the object more closely. Initially, he thought it was a piece of wood or a large rock, but then he thought maybe it was a mannequin. However, that didn't sit quite right either, as the angle of the head and neck of a mannequin wouldn't be at the angle it was, and the way the left arm was bent up across the chest didn't look how a mannequin's arm would bend.

He stared hard down into the murkiness and came to the conclusion that it might be a dead person. Taking out his mobile phone, he called 000. A female operator answered and Tae said, 'I think I just saw a dead body in the water'.

He then provided quite a bit of detail, which proved helpful, as police arrived at the scene a short time later. Tae pointed out the body and a female officer walked him over to a wooden bench nearby to take down the particulars of his story. More police arrived, including detectives from Eastwood, Chatswood crime scene operatives and personnel from Police Rescue. A number of photographs were taken before the corpse was removed from the creek and conveyed to the Glebe mortuary by the Government Contractors, Statewide Mortuary Transfers.

At 4 pm in the afternoon, ZhiYing Zang formally identified the body as that of her grandson, Lin Lee.

The post-mortem examination was carried out at 9 am on 23 October by forensic pathologist Dr Lillian Schwartz, in the presence of Deborah Sayers, the autopsy assistant. In summary, Dr Schwartz opined that at autopsy, bruising was present over the anterior aspect of both shins. No other injuries were noted on external examination of the body. The hands and feet showed changes characteristic of prolonged water immersion. Adhesions were noted in the right chest cavity. Upon microscopic examination, the liver showed congestion of the central zones. Other tissues showed no obvious abnormalities. The toxicological analysis of the post-mortem blood specimen detected a small amount of alcohol which may have caused a slight physiological impairment. In addition, the blood specimen detected a toxic level of quetiapine.

A blood sample taken from Lin Li at the post-mortem was found to have present quetiapine 3.3 milligrams per litre and alcohol 0.023 grams per decilitre (100 millilitres) of blood.

I was aware that quetiapine is a dibenzothiazepine-type anti-psychotic which is available under the trade name 'Seroquel'. The drug is used to treat the symptoms of schizophrenia or bipolar disorder and various other mental disorders. The blood concentration of quetiapine was well outside the therapeutic range (0.195 - 0.632 µg/ml or mg/L) and indicates that [the deceased] had ingested a large dosage of the drug. However, whilst the drug level is within the toxic range it is unlikely by itself, to have taken his life.

Further, quetiapine is available as the fumarate salt in tablets of 25, 100 and 200 milligrams (mg) for oral administration. Daily doses in adults are usually 300 – 450 mg (range 150 – 750 mg/day). The most common side effect of quetiapine is somnolence (sleepiness). Other common side effects include hypertension, dizziness, dry mouth and dyspepsia (upset stomach). The drug has been abused for its euphoric properties. Quetiapine may exhibit post-mortem redistribution with heart/femoral blood level ratios averaging 1.3 (range 0.6 – 2.6), this becomes greater with increasing decomposition of the body. Additionally, a small amount of alcohol was detected in the [deceased's] blood. This was most likely due microbial/yeast fermentation of the glucose in the deceased's blood as his body was showing signs of decomposition.

I concluded, relying on the information supplied, that at the time of the incident, given the amount of quetiapine in his blood, [the deceased's] ability to save himself once immersed in the water, would have been compromised.

It's probable that Lin Lee, intoxicated with quetiapine, had been walking along Terry's Creek bushwalk, seeking solitude and, on reaching the pedestrian footbridge, he'd most likely lost his balance and fallen into the dark waters below.

A subsequent inquest found that it was an accidental death, with the excessive consumption of quetiapine most likely being a contributing factor to his drowning death.

29

'Hey, Mum, I can fly!' The Tragic Death of a Star Student

'Don't try to fly before you have wings.'
~ French Proverb

Killara is an affluent suburb on the Upper North Shore of Sydney, New South Wales. Located fourteen kilometres north-west of the Sydney central business district, the word 'killara' is aboriginal for 'permanent' or 'always there'. Killara is home to two high ranking public primary schools - Killara Public School and Beaumont Road Public School - as well as Killara High School, which is recognised as one of the top performing non-selective government secondary schools in the state.

This case involves a very promising teenage boy who attended Killara High. His name was Yi-Heng Kwan. Aged seventeen, he was in his final year, studying for his Higher School Certificate (HSC). Besides being a popular and likeable teenager, he was one of the school's brightest students and could speak six languages fluently. He was born in Taiwan, but his family moved to Singapore and then Australia. With Singapore being a bilingual country, the English language became second nature to him, and when the Kwan family arrived in Australia, Yi-Heng soon learnt that he had to work hard at his studies to get ahead and achieve his ambitions of becoming a lawyer or a doctor. Which one was almost immaterial, as he had the potential to 'fly' in whichever career he chose.

But the pressures of the HSC and the need to succeed were great. Any helpful prop would ease the pressure. Yi-Heng just wanted something to stimulate him sufficiently to get through another night of study. A friend at school, Tzu-Yang Fang, was reputed to have a supply of a drug which was believed to aid studying. Perhaps that was the answer to Yi-Heng's prayers. And at only $1.50 per tab, it was very cheap.

On 5 June, 2013, Yi-Heng was collected from school, along with his younger sister, Michelle, who was fourteen years old. His mother and sister planned to do some shopping before returning to their apartment, so they dropped off Yi-Heng, who asked them to pick up some sushi for dinner. While they were gone, he took a tab and began studying. But when his mother and sister returned an hour or so later, they found him in a psychotic state. He had no appetite for the sushi and, after a very rapid greeting, he took off to his room and started to smash bottles on the floor. His mother told him in no uncertain terms to desist and clean up the mess, whereupon he walked out of his room and vomited. Due to the synthetic psychosis that possessed him, he was incapable of doing what his mother wanted, and he told her that he was sorry, but he'd taken something. His mother managed to get him into the shower, and when he was dry, to put on some clean clothes, which he then took off and wouldn't put back on. She then persuaded him to settle down a little and watch television, but after a little while, he cried out, 'I want to fly, I want to fly'.

Before anyone could stop him, he ran to the balcony, where an intense stand-off occurred, with his mother and sister struggling to stop him climbing over the edge. For more than an hour they tried to reason with the naked, increasingly psychotic young man, and the commotion attracted the attention of neighbours in the apartment complex. His mother grabbed him by the foot whilst his sister grabbed him by the arm. Out of the blue, he bit his sister, causing her to release her grip, and he launched himself over the balcony, striking the pavement three stories below.

He sustained extensive head injuries and subsequently died at the scene.

Police later said that they knew it was an NBOM-e product, most likely the drug 25I-NBOMe, that he'd ingested prior to his death.

Traditionally, drugs of abuse have come mainly from plant products such as cannabis *(Cannabis sativa),* opium poppies *(Papaver somniferum),* cocaine *(Erythroxylon coca),* hallucinogenic mushrooms *(Psilocybe cubenis)* and peyote cactus *(Lophophore williamsii)* which contains the hallucinogen, mescaline. Today, however, many drugs of abuse which are structurally and pharmacologically similar to designated controlled substances are produced in clandestine laboratories. Furthermore, these drugs do not appear themselves to be controlled substances. They have been described as so-called legal highs. The term 'designer drug' was first used by law enforcement agencies in the 1980s, and has since gained widespread use. These drugs were created to get around existing drug laws, usually by preparing analogues or derivatives of existing drugs by modifying their chemical structure to varying degrees.

In some cases, the structural modification increases the potency of the drug. This was the situation with NBOM-e drugs. NBOM-e or N-Bomb drugs (a street name derived from the chemical abbreviation) are a new class of hallucinogenic stimulants derived from a relatively old class of phenylalkylamine drugs: the so-called, 2C- x series of drugs. For example, 2C-I is a substituted analogue of mescaline, with the halogen, iodine, substituted for the 4-methoxy group, producing 4-Iodo-2, 5-dimethoxy-4-phenethylamine.

4-Iodo-2, 5-dimethoxy-4-phenethylamine or 2, 5-dimethoxy-4iodophen-ethylamine (also known as 2C-I, Smiles, 4-iodo- 2, 5-DMPEA) is a synthetic hallucinogen with a greater potency than mescaline and properties similar to LSD.

Smiles has been used and abused orally as tablets and snorted in its powder form. At a dosage of approximately five milligrams orally, the user becomes passive and relaxed. There is euphoria with increased body awareness and enhanced receptiveness of visual, auditory, olfactory and tactile sensations similar to ecstasy. Oral doses of ten to twenty-five milligrams produce stimulant effects and cause a full intoxicated state. Doses in the range of twenty to thirty milligrams produce LSD-like hallucinations. Dosages greater than fifty milligrams have produced very fearful hallucinations and morbid delusions. The effects of the drug after ingestion begin to occur after ten to twenty minutes, peaking at between one to two hours, and they can last for anything from four to twelve hours. The unpleasant physical side-effects included muscle tension, overstimulation, hallucinations, nausea, seizures and vomiting. The N-Bomb drug, 25I-NBOMe - the drug that Yi-Heng took - is derived from 2C-I. 25I-NBOMe is synthesised by reacting the drug 2-methoxybenzaldehyde (MeOB) with the amine nitrogen on the phenethylamine backbone. This substitution substantially increases the potency of the drug's activity and also the drug's unpleasant side effects. Some of these symptoms were experienced by Yi-Heng before his ill-fated 'flight'.

Another N-Bomb drug derived from an 'old' drug is Nexus or 2C-B.

4-Bromo-2, 5-dimethoxyphenethylamine (also known as 2C-B, 4-bromo-2,5-DMPEA and Nexus) is a synthetic hallucinogen. The 'old' drug used to be taken mainly for its hallucinogenic effects as a club drug on the rave culture and circuit party scenes before being banned. 2C-I took its place. Nexus has been used and abused orally in tablet or capsule forms, or snorted in its powder guise. It has a similar effect on the user to Smiles: at a dosage of approximately four milligrams orally, the user becomes passive and relaxed. There is euphoria with increased body awareness and enhanced receptiveness of visual, auditory, olfactory and tactile sensations similar to ecstasy. Oral doses of eight to ten milligrams produce stimulant effects and cause a full intoxicated state. Doses in the range of twenty to forty milligrams produce LSD-like hallucinations. Dosages greater than fifty milligrams have produced very fearful hallucinations and morbid delusions. The effects of the drug after ingestion begin to occur after twenty to thirty minutes, peaking at between one and a half to two hours, and the effects can last for six to eight hours.

25B-NBOMe (N-Bomb, New Nexus) is derived from 2C-B and is synthesised by reacting the drug 2-methoxybenzaldehyde (MeOB) with the amine nitrogen on the phenethylamine backbone. This substitution also substantially increases the potency of the drug's activity, resulting in a very potent hallucinogen with pharmacological active doses in the microgram range (250 - 500µg), which puts the drug into the LSD range. However, the dosages vary from person to person and are subjective.

Women sadly are affected by it more than men, while a person's weight also matters. Just as LSD also builds up a tolerance very fast, meaning that more is needed next time to reach the same effect again, so the same applies to the very potent 2C-x synthetics.

Unfortunately for Yi-Heng Kwan, he ingested this very potent drug and became its latest victim at the time.

At the inquest, it was obvious from the outset how popular he'd been, as friends and family members openly wept during proceedings, necessitating a brief adjournment so they could compose themselves. The coroner found that Yi-Heng's death was caused by misadventure. In other words, it was an accidental death.

It was clear that the bizarre behaviour he'd exhibited on the balcony of his family's apartment in Killara and the desire to 'fly' had been very much out of character, and had been almost certainly due to the effects of a very potent hallucinogen, N-Bomb or 25I-NOBMe.

Later on, in Parramatta Local Court, on 14 April 2014, nineteen-year-old Tzu-Yang Fang, who sold Yi-Heng the drug-laced tab, pleaded not guilty to one count of supplying a prohibited drug to his classmate, and went free because he'd been charged with selling LSD, which he hadn't done.

Toxicologists in the 1980s predicted that the future drugs of abuse would be synthetics rather than plant products. The drugs would be synthesised from readily available chemicals, and might be derivatives of pharmaceuticals and would be very potent, and often very selective in their action. In addition, they would be marketed very cleverly.

That prediction has proved to be remarkably accurate.

These so-called designer drugs now present the new face of drug abuse, resulting in very real challenges to clinicians, treatment providers, emergency departments, laboratories, prosecutors, police, poison control centres, workplace screening, families and legislators. In order to prevent further deaths like Yi-Heng Kwan from this new generation of drugs and the dreadful knock-on effects to society, the Justice Minister, Michael Keenan, unveiled new laws designed to end the booming synthetic drug industry and force importers to prove they have legitimate use.

He said, 'These drugs are often marketed as safe and credible alternatives to illicit drugs such as LSD. Yet, tragically, we have learned too many times through death or injury to people, especially young people, that this is not the case and they are extremely dangerous. There's nothing synthetic about the damage these drugs cause. They are not harmless. They are not safe. They have deadly consequences. We do not want a market for this misery in Australia'.

The traditional approach was to list the various drugs under the Drugs Misuse and Trafficking Act (DMT Act) and ban them, including precursors that are used to make them. However, the concern was that importers would make new types of synthetic drugs with a slightly different chemical structure - and they did!

That loophole was closed by adding additional drugs to the DMT Act and including the analogue clause (Schedule 1) to counteract any modifications. Hopefully, it will help prevent future tragic cases like Yi-Heng Kwan.

But so long as young people are willing to experiment with drugs of dubious toxicological properties and origin, along with huge profits to be made by the manufacturers and distributors, causalities will continue to occur.

And so, the battle continues, as illustrated in the next story.

30

An 'Unbearable High': A Death by 'Bath Salts'

'If you drink much from a bottle marked "poison", it is almost certain to disagree with you, sooner or later.'

~ **_Lewis Carroll,_** *Alice through the Looking Glass*

Alpha-pyrrolidinovalero-phenone or -PVP (alpha-PVP) is a synthetic psychoactive drug which has stimulant effects on both the central nervous system (CNS) and on the cardiovascular system. Depending on upon the dosage, it can result in euphoria, social empathy, heightened appreciation of music and visual stimuli and increased alertness and elevated mood – which are the main reasons the drug is used recreationally.

It's known by various street names, including Plant Food, or the more popular Bath Salts, and quite often carries a disclaimer stating that it isn't for human consumption to get around state and federal laws. However, a number of new amendments to the existing Drug Misuse and Trafficking Act (1985) Schedule

1 have been made to address the problem of such drug derivatives, and as such, alpha-PVP is considered to be a structural modification of methcathinone through the addition of a heterocyclic ring structure to a carbon. Having the same constituent groups, the similarity in structure is obvious. In other words, being a structural derivative of an already existing banned substance, the drug now falls under the Drug Misuse and Trafficking Law.

But more importantly, from the potential user's point of view, the drug isn't subject to the various quality and toxicology considerations given to pharmacy drugs and displays various adverse effects, which are very important. Those include increased heart rate, hypertension (raised blood pressure), vasoconstriction, sweating, loss of appetite, hyponatremia (low sodium in the blood), anxiety, paranoia, hyperthermia (elevated body temperature) and renal failure (the kidneys are adversely affected).

Given these latter effects, alongside the uncertainty of dosage levels required to obtain even minimal gain, why do people take the risks of using the product? Fortunately, not all people are affected in the same way. Most users experience the desired pleasurable high, a euphoric-type of experience, which is much sought after, and that in turn leads to further sales. The product used to 'fly off the shelves' in adult shops, tobacconists and online suppliers, so it must have been good, with even alleged wanted fugitive and software multimillionaire John McAfee being linked in online comments saying he was a 'huge fan'.

Long-distance truck driver Glenn Punch, aged forty-four, and his de facto wife Rachael Hickel, aged forty-two, were an average, affectionate, fun-loving couple. On Friday, 19 October 2012, they stopped by an adult shop, Nauti & Nice, in Thornton – a suburb of Newcastle, New South Wales – and purchased a bag of a nondescript white powder called Smokin' Slurry Scrubba, which was said to have effects similar to Speed. The pack was labelled 'not for human consumption', but was marketed online and in various forums as a legal high. The shop assistant assured them that the products they sold were all legal, but added, 'with the sensation you get from an illegal drug'. Glenn and Rachael took the drug back to the motel in which they were staying, where Glenn mixed the powder with some water and injected himself with the substance.

Very quickly his behaviour changed, becoming strange and out of character, and he took off all his clothes. Observing the disturbing effects it was having on her partner, Rachel flushed the remainder of the drug down the toilet. However, despite that occurrence, they bought Smokin' Slurry Scrubba on several more occasions that weekend, each time experiencing the same strange hallucinatory effects. Glenn would inject himself and his partner, and then strip off his clothing. From eyewitness accounts, he displayed paranoid and bizarre behaviour over a number of hours. Rachael also experienced strange effects, which included hallucinations, such as seeing people inside the house with their hands waving, feeling really hot, her heart racing and feeling dehydrated.

Incredibly, during the afternoon of Sunday, 21 October, they bought some more Smokin' Slurry Scrubba powder from Nauti & Nice, although it was from a different outlet - the one in Rutherford, Newcastle. One can only speculate why after their experience with the purchase from the Thornton store, but perhaps their subsequent purchases from other places led them to believe that they'd just been unlucky and bought from a bad batch. Anyway, after making the purchase and returning to his rig (truck), Glenn again mixed the drug with some water and injected both himself and Rachael. It was time to have fun. However, the drug that he'd purchased proved to be quite different from the one he'd bought in Thornton. The drug mixture was the colour of tan not clear as it had been with the previous purchases.

Rachael suddenly overbalanced and fell out of the rig, hitting the road and suffering head injuries. Bloodied and naked from the waist upwards, she staggered down the highway in a very erratic manner, covering a fair distance before being stopped and cared for by passing motorists, who called for an ambulance which took her to hospital.

In the meantime, Glenn had once again removed all his clothing and fallen out of the rig after her, but he'd gone stumbling and zigzagging in the opposite direction, towards a nearby shipping yard belonging to Forgacs, a ship building company. Amazingly, he managed to scale the eight foot high (2.44 metres) perimeter security fence, which was topped by barbed wire, and climb over into the yard where he ran about maniacally before charging into an old administration building. Security guard Vincent Hagens notified the police and, after seeing Punch smash a glass exit door with an aluminium ladder, went after him. Hagens grabbed Punch and a struggle ensued, with Punch displaying extraordinary strength. At first it appeared that Punch was getting the better of Hagens, even though they were of similar weight and height, but the struggle continued, with the two combatants falling down a flight of stairs and Hagens suffering a bite to his wrist. Fortunately fellow employee Luke Riding came to help his colleague.

They eventually managed to hold Punch to the ground by using their knees and holding his arms, but still he struggled, showing super strength. Then he started to foam at the mouth. A moment later, he suddenly stopped struggling and went limp. His breathing also appeared to have stopped. Alarmed, Riding went for medical help just as the police arrived. They began CPR, which was continued until the paramedics could take over. Punch was taken to Calvary Mater Hospital, but he never regained consciousness. He was later transferred to the intensive care unit of the Prince of Wales Hospital, Randwick, where he died after life support was discontinued on 23 October.

A number of blood samples were taken from Punch's body at an ante-mortem (whilst in hospital) and at the post-mortem for toxicological examination, along with a number of resealable plastic bags containing a crystalline powder found in his truck.

The initial blood samples only showed the presence of lignocaine (less than 0.2 milligrams per litre), morphine (free) 0.02 milligrams per litre and midazolam 0.03 milligrams per litre.

Lignocaine is used as a local anaesthetic and for the treatment of life-threatening ventricular arrhythmias, while midazolam is used as a short-acting sleep-inducing agent for conscious sedation and induction of anaesthesia. It was most likely given to Punch to treat his agitation. The morphine present in his blood sample was at about the therapeutic level, indicating a moderate ingestion of the drug. An examination of his medical records showed those drugs to be part of the medical treatment regimen utilised to save Punch's life.

So what caused his demise?

Attention turned to the contents of the plastic bags found in his possession. They were analysed and found to contain alpha-pyrrolidinovalero-phenone (or alpha-PVP). With that knowledge, it seemed likely, given Punch's symptoms before being conveyed to hospital, that that drug was most likely present in his blood samples. Using a sensitive technique known as selective-ion monitoring the blood samples were re-examined and, sure enough, both the ante-mortem and post-mortem blood samples were found to contain alpha-PVP.

It was the culprit drug, and one which can produce symptoms that include psychosis, paranoia, violence, agitation, hallucinations, increased body temperature and confusion, which can sometimes last for days depending on the dose. Both Glenn Punch and Rachael Hickel experienced some of these symptoms in varying degrees. However, it is the tachycardia and arrhythmias, along with hyperthermia (elevated body temperature) that can result in death if not rapidly treated.

An inquest took place at Glebe Coroner's Court, from 8 -10 October, 2013, before Magistrate Mary Jerram, the NSW state coroner. At the centre of the enquiry were three main issues: the cause of Glenn Punch's death, the legality of Smokin' Slurry Scrubba, which had been found to contain alpha-PVP and had been the drug found in Glenn Punch's system, and whether there should be any consideration of any referral to the Director of Public Prosecutions under section 78 of the 2009 Coroners Act.

As to the cause of death of Glenn Punch, forensic pathologist Dr Lillian Schwartz stated in her initial report that the cause was 'complications of drug toxicity, most likely a stimulant of the amphetamine family and cerebellar tonsillar herniation'.

After receiving the supplementary analyst's certificate, I stated in my report, 'Alpha-PVP is a synthetic psychoactive drug with central nervous system (CNS) stimulant effects which functions as a noradrenaline (norepinephrine) – dopamine reuptake inhibitor (NDRI). As such, it has stimulatory effects on the CNS and cardiovascular system which result in the following effects - euphoria, social empathy, heightened appreciation of music and visual stimuli, increased alertness and elevated mood.

‘However, adverse reactions to alpha-PVP include increased heart rate, hypertension (raised blood pressure), vasoconstriction, sweating, loss of appetite, hyponatremia (low sodium in the blood), anxiety, paranoia, hyperthermia (elevated body temperature) and renal failure. Some of these symptoms were displayed by Mr Punch on admission to hospital including hyperthermia (39 degrees Celsius) and low sodium (hyponatremia).

‘Alpha-PVP is a potent inhibitor of dopamine and noradrenaline (norepinephrine) transport, but is a relatively poor inhibitor of serotonin transport which may account for its psychological effects. However, this depends upon the dosage ingested and the regimen followed (namely, whether single or multiple doses are ingested).’

I concluded, based on my specialised knowledge and relying on the information supplied, that I was of the opinion that given Mr. Punch’s symptoms (including cerebellar tonsillar herniation) and the presence of alpha-PVP in his blood, that this drug was most likely the cause of his death.

Dr Schwartz reached a similar conclusion after the supplementary report had been received, stating the cause of death was ‘Alpha-pyrro-lidino-pentio-phenone Toxicity’ (Alpha PVP).

Both Dr Schwartz and I gave concurrent evidence (a procedure known as ‘hot-tubbing’), along with three other experts, Dr Johan Duflou (Senior Forensic Pathologist at Glebe), Professor Alison Jones, a toxicologist and Professor Iain McGregor, a neuropharmacologist. Dr Duflou was unable to determine the exact cause of death and considered that restraint asphyxia (or positional asphyxia) may have occurred while Punch was being restrained by the security guards. However, he did state that it was most likely that if Punch hadn’t consumed alpha-PVP, he wouldn’t have died. Professor Jones disagreed that positional asphyxia was a possible cause of death, and Professor McGregor agreed with him. I thought the issue was irrelevant. An important point raised by Professor Jones was the fact Punch had injected the drug, thus raising the toxicity greatly because a larger dose had entered his system, leading to an ‘outburst of adrenalin’, which in turn had resulted in cardiac arrhythmia and then cerebral oedema (a build-up of fluid in the brain).

Eventually, we all agreed that alpha-PVP had contributed to Punch's death.

The next issue was the legality of the sale of those synthetic drugs.

While the Smokin' Slurry Scrubba had been found to contain alpha-PVP and the same drug had been found in Punch's system at the time of his death, alpha-PVP wasn't specifically listed in Schedule 1 of the Drug Misuse and Trafficking Act (DMTA). However, I pointed out to the court that due to its psychotropic properties and chemical structure, alpha-PVP was captured by the analogue provisions of the Act, and therefore illegal by virtue of the drug being an analogue of methcathinone, a substance listed at that time in the DMTA, under Schedule 1.

The next issue was whether there should be any consideration of any referral to the Director of Public Prosecutions under section 78 of the 2009 Coroners Act relating to the drug alpha-PVP. However, just before the inquest into the death of Glenn Punch commenced, a teenager died after jumping off a balcony following the consumption of a synthetic drug (see previous story), which resulted in legislative changes outlawing psychoactive substances and adding alpha PVP to Schedule I of the DMTA. Therefore, it was no longer necessary for the court to consider making recommendations under Section 82 of the Coroner's Act relating to those drugs, as they were, by then, prohibited.

However, in spite of that, distributors, retailers and consumers of those synthetic drugs still believed them to be legal. In particular, 'Nauti and Nice' had apparently sought legal advice from a company called Northside Law about selling the drugs. Letters addressed to the distributing company stated that 'there was no prohibition on the sale, possession or use of a product called Smoking Slurry, "Hoe", whose active substance was alpha-PVP'. Mr Mathew Wynn, the manager of Nauti and Nice, said that he relied on those letters to sell the drugs, maintaining that he thought they were legal highs. The principal solicitor of Northside Law, Mr David Ross, gave evidence which suggested that because he hadn't seen the word alpha-PVP in the Schedule of the Act, he'd assumed that it wasn't proscribed, and had produced letters based on that belief. When questioned by Peter Hamill SC, of the Crown Solicitor's Office and assisting coroner, about alpha-PV –, a substance that is an analogue to a listed substance – Mr Ross admitted he didn't fully understand the provisions for analogues in the drugs legislation, saying, 'It's very difficult to understand what an analogue means. It's very difficult to put your finger on how that would affect a client in regards to criminal statute. I didn't think the word analogue conveyed a meaning that was intended to apply to the substance'.

Peter Hamill asked if Mr Ross had read the analogue provisions.

He replied in the affirmative.

Hamill then posed a further question, 'Did that give you any idea as to what an analogue meant?'

Mr Ross replied, 'Not to my recollection'.

Peter Hamill had earlier addressed the inquest, saying that Glenn Punch, Rachael Hickel, the distributors and owners of the Nauti and Nice adult shop (where the dangerous drug had been sold) were under the mistaken belief that the drug was legal.

The shop assistants working at the Nauti and Nice shops said that while the packets of drugs were marked 'not for human use', they were well aware that they were being bought to be consumed. And the profits were huge; some stores made up to $7000 daily, with the drugs forming about eighty per cent of their sales. One of the shopkeepers openly admitted to having snorted and drunk Scrubba, as well as taking the drug intravenously. He described the effects from intravenous use as 'surprising', with effects far stronger than amphetamines, which he apparently used on a regular basis. He told the court, 'I can't believe this is legal'.

However, he also admitted he never discussed the legality of the products or the accompanying health risks with his employers because, 'I didn't want them to know I was using the product'.

One of the female workers said she'd worked at Nauti and Nice for about three years, and that while she herself never used the drugs, she'd seen manic behaviour in some customers who did. She related the tale of one female customer who used Smokin' Slurry, who asked her if she could 'eat her face' before going outside and eating from a dead animal that was on the road!

For some individuals, the drug clearly has unpredictable effects. This, together with its psychotropic effects and the varying potency of batches presented for sale, makes it one of a number of synthetic drugs that are very dangerous for consumers.

As Peter Hamill, SC, said, 'The drug clearly had psychotropic effects. The substance wasn't legal. The troubling thing is that it appears there was real confusion over that … and it seems it was utterly unregulated'.

After hearing evidence from a number of other witnesses, the coroner made her formal finding: 'Glenn Punch died at 8.23 am on October 23, 2012 at the Prince of Wales Hospital, Randwick, NSW of cardiac arrest and cerebral oedema consequent upon ingestion of a synthetic drug known as Smokin' Slurry or Scrubba, containing the chemical Alpha PVP, and possibly associated with his being restrained'.

So much for Glenn Punch, but what happened to his de facto wife Rachael Hickel?

I'm afraid that as tragic as Glenn Punch's demise was, it's arguable he got the better of the deal. Poor Rachael suffered from severe hallucinations for the next six months. She was said to have described the effects as being like 'as if I was driving in my car at night time. I would have the interior light on because (I'd see) people coming out of the boot trying to get me'. Following that, her hallucinations became so intense that she lost contact with reality and didn't even believe Glenn Punch had died. She said, 'I thought it was all fake, even at the funeral'.

The drug seriously affected her brain chemistry, and the prognosis doesn't look good for her. Sadly, it is possible she could now wind up in a mental institution.

These drugs, and their derivatives, are very dangerous.

Alpha-PVP and other stimulants have since been outlawed following sweeping changes to synthetic drug legislation in New South Wales. This is probably of cold comfort to both Rachael, who not only lost a friend and lover to a perilous and unregulated drug but also now struggles to know what day of the week it is, and to the Kwan family (see previous story) who lost a son to the effects of another synthetic amphetamine, which also scrambled the brain chemistry with unpredictable effects.

Drug manufacturers now routinely alter compounds, and a new drug hits the streets every week in an attempt to get around state and national laws, with suppliers paying solicitors to argue that they're legal. It's now become a situation where the prosecution must prove that the drugs have a chemical structure and intended pharmacological effect that is 'substantially similar' to the scheduled dangerous drugs. Fortunately, the drug legislation in Australia was drafted by some very clever people, particularly under the Schedule 1 provisions, and allows for alterations in the molecular structure of drugs. However, potential users should be aware of the unpredictable side effects of these new so-called designer drugs and their possible long-term effects – if they survive…

About the Author

Sitting Bull, (c. 1831-1890) a famous Native American Indian Sioux chief once said *"Do not let the poisons of the world pull you from your path."* Curiously, the opposite was true for Dr William J. Allender. His path has led him to many poisons (and drug) cases and the need to help various authorities to prosecute the villains who chose to use them in their nefarious and evil deeds.

As a forensic toxicologist, Dr Allender (or 'Dr Bill') has been called to give expert witness evidence in a number of very high profile cases involving drug overdoses and poisons (including pesticides), in which those substances have been used in suicides and murder. He has also given evidence in coronial matters that have become so emotional that the court has had to be adjourned for members of the family to compose themselves. As for many other cases, a number stand out due to the unusual circumstances, one involving a drug-affected young man who was killed on Sydney Harbour Bridge, ('A Case of MDMA Madness') another where a body was disposed of into a wheelie bin ('The Body in the Wheelie Bin Murder'), an evil pair who spiked the drinks of their dates to carry out their crimes ('Drink Spiking: A Two Man Crime Wave') and the sad case of Dianne Brimble who went on a well- deserved cruise, only to wind up dead from a drug over-dose ('Death on the High Seas..'), to name but a few.

Acknowledgements

I would like to thank my former colleagues at the Clinical Forensic Medicine Unit, police officers (both New South Wales and Australian Federal Police) and folk at the Department of Public Prosecution I had the privilege to work with and to discuss the many case matters we had to deal with as a team. In particular, I wish to thank Detective Sergeant Barry Fay (retired) and his former colleague, Detective Superintendent Ron Stephenson (sadly deceased) who inspired me to write these stories.

I wish to also acknowledge Roy Matoir, who sorted my technical/scientific prose from my many stories into more readable form. For that I thank him for his efforts.

Thank you to my wonderful family and close friends, whose encouragement helped make this book possible.

My thanks to my publisher, Lesley Pagett, for her skills and understanding, it was a pleasure working with you. I'd like to also thank Elise James, my editor, for her advice and attention to detail, throughout the editing process. To the wonderful team at New Holland books, I can't thank you enough. It has been a pleasure to work with you all.

First published in 2019 by New Holland Publishers
Sydney • Auckland

Level 1, 178 Fox Valley Road, Wahroonga, NSW 2076, Australia
5/39 Woodside Ave, Northcote, Auckland 0627, New Zealand

newhollandpublishers.com

A record of this book is held at the the National Library of Australia.

ISBN 9781760791490

Group Managing Director: Fiona Schultz
Publisher: Lesley Pagett
Project Editor: Elise James
Designer Front Cover: Andrew Davies
Designer: Yolanda La Gorcé
Production Director: Arlene Gippert

10 9 8 7 6 5 4 3 2 1

Keep up with New Holland Publishers:

NewHollandPublishers

@newhollandpublishers